A Mouth Full of Poison

THE TRUTH ABOUT MERCURY AMALGAM FILLINGS

D0311348

BY DR. MYRON WENTZ

A Mouth Full of Poison

TABLE OF CONTENTS

9   FOREWORD

13   INTRODUCTION

17   CHAPTER 1: THE HISTORY OF THE MERCURY AMALGAM WARS

29   CHAPTER 2: MERCURY, MERCURY EVERYWHERE

37   CHAPTER 3: THE POISONOUS NATURE OF MERCURY

49   CHAPTER 4: REGULATORY STANDARDS

53   CHAPTER 5: LEGISLATIVE & REGULATORY INITIATIVES

61   CHAPTER 6: YOUR MOUTH—A TOXIC RESERVOIR

71   CHAPTER 7: INTO THE MOUTHS OF BABES

83   CHAPTER 8: MECHANISMS OF MERCURY TOXICITY

93   CHAPTER 9: DETOXIFICATION MECHANISMS

101   CHAPTER 10: THE DENTAL OFFICE—A HAZARDOUS WORKPLACE

107   CHAPTER 11: VARIATIONS IN MERCURY EXPOSURE

119   CHAPTER 12: ASSESSING YOUR MERCURY RISK

137   CHAPTER 13: WHAT'S NEXT FOR YOU?

145   CHAPTER 14: HEALTH BENEFITS OF REMOVING MERCURY FROM THE BODY

157   CHAPTER 15: ON THE FIRING LINE

165   ON A PERSONAL NOTE

167   REFERENCES

TABLES

32 TABLE 2-1: INDUSTRIAL USES OF MERCURY

34 TABLE 2-2: ESTIMATED DAILY INTAKE & RETENTION OF MERCURY

41 TABLE 3-1: COMMON SYMPTOMS OF CHRONIC MERCURY POISONING

42 TABLE 3-2: DISEASES RELATED TO MERCURY POISONING

45 TABLE 3-3: COMMON ALLERGY SYMPTOMS

46 TABLE 3-4: DISEASES AGGRAVATED BY ALLERGY TO METALS

68 TABLE 6-1: STIMULATION OF AMALGAM FILLINGS

98 TABLE 9-1: NUTRIENTS INVOLVED IN GLUTATHIONE METABOLISM

112 TABLE 11-1: COMPOSITION OF DENTAL AMALGAM (BY PERCENT)

130 TABLE 12-1: COMMON SYMPTOMS OF CHRONIC MERCURY POISONING

131 TABLE 12-2: DISEASES RELATED TO MERCURY POISONING

132 TABLE 12-3: INDUSTRIAL USE OF MERCURY

134 TABLE 12-4: ADDING THE POINTS

135 TABLE 12-5: RISK CATEGORIES

138 TABLE 13-1: SERVICES OFFERED BY MERCURY-FREE DENTISTS

146 TABLE 14-1: SYMPTOM IMPROVEMENT AFTER AMALGAM REMOVAL

FOREWORD

Having had the pleasure of working closely with Dr. Myron Wentz on a number of health related projects, I was pleased to act as a consultant on his book and honored when he asked me to write the foreword. I know Dr. Wentz both professionally and as a friend. Over the years, I have come to appreciate what an exceptional human being he is: a man of vision and action who not only recognizes a problem when he sees it but is also able to create a solution.

In 1977, through his company, Gull Laboratories, Dr. Wentz researched and developed several diagnostic assays, including the analytical test, used around the world today, for the Epstein-Barr virus. The clinical assay has prevented immeasurable suffering and financial hardship by allowing early detection and treatment of this debilitating virus. Later, Dr. Wentz founded USANA, a state-of-the-art manufacturer of pharmaceutical-grade nutritional supplements. USANA products are now listed in the prominent *Physician's Desk Reference* (PDR) and have recently been rated in the *Comparative Guide to Nutritional Supplements* as the best vitamin supplements in North America. Today, USANA products are sold worldwide.

After establishing USANA in 1992, Dr. Wentz turned his focus to the creation of a world-class center for holistic healing. *Sanoviv Medical Institute* is a fully accredited, leading-edge medical facility and the only one in the western hemisphere that bridges the gap between the medical and dental worlds. The Sanoviv philosophy reflects Dr. Wentz's personal belief that the human body has the power to heal itself, when given the proper environment and relieved of its toxic burden. Sanoviv is a remarkable haven that challenges conventional medicine, taking the best that science has to offer and blending it with the wisdom of Mother Nature.

In 2001, Dr. Wentz and USANA joined the Children's Hunger Fund in providing nutritional supplements to impoverished children throughout the world. Through the Children's Hunger Fund Care Package Program, USANA employees and associates have adopted entire families, providing them with monthly shipments of nutritious food, supplements, clothing, hygiene products, toys, and other items much needed to improve their lives. The results have been phenomenal: thousands of children throughout the world are now benefiting from Dr. Wentz's vision and the compassion and support of USANA's worldwide family. The partnership with the Children's Hunger Fund is helping to make Dr. Wentz's dream of "a world free from pain and suffering" become a reality.

On a personal level, I see Dr. Wentz as a combination of Jonas Salk, Albert Schweitzer, and Linus Pauling. It takes the creative genius of a Jonas Salk to find solutions to such major health challenges as chronic mercury poisoning. It takes the dedication, sincerity and devotion of an Albert Schweitzer to work tirelessly for the betterment of humankind, and it takes the commitment of a Linus Pauling to persevere against ignorance and enormous peer pressure in order to succeed where others have failed.

Now that you know something about Myron Wentz, let me tell you why I am so excited about what he is doing for hundreds of millions of people who have mercury amalgam fillings. I know of no other chronic health issue that is more important than the poisonous effects of mercury amalgam. As a dental professional, I have remained adamantly opposed to them for over 30 years, and I thoroughly understand how harmful these toxic fillings are to overall health. When Dr. Wentz first discussed his ideas for this book with me, I was impressed with his grasp of the issues. Now, in *A Mouth Full of Poison* he addresses the mercury amalgam issue with honesty, thoroughness, and clarity.

For over 160 years, the dental industry has deliberately confused the public and papered over the very real hazards of mercury amalgam. Dr. Wentz has finally shone the light of scientific truth on this controversial subject. His presentation of the case against amalgam fillings is a wakeup call that promises to transform how we view this matter. In presenting his findings, Dr. Wentz has systematically laid to waste the dental profession's claims of safety, and has done so in a scientifically rigorous way that everyone can understand. Anyone who has been confused and uncertain about this issue will be shocked at the revelations. From layperson to professional, anyone who truly cares about their health or the health of their patients will benefit immensely from this insightful book.

I am thrilled that a leader has emerged to oppose the use of these toxic fillings. It takes an individual of Dr. Wentz's stature and dedication—one who understands and can communicate the scientific nuances of the issue—to put forth the case to have mercury amalgam fillings forever banned. With Dr. Wentz on the front line, there is no doubt in my mind that the battle against these fillings will finally be won.

This book is a powerful testimony to the hidden dangers of chronic mercury toxicity. It is an essential read for everyone who has been or could be exposed to amalgam fillings, especially mothers and mothers-to-be. It is for everyone who has symptoms of mercury poisoning and who wants to know how these fillings have affected their health and what they can do about it. And it is for everyone who wants to prevent future health problems related to mercury amalgams, both for themselves and their families.

If you have ever been confused about the controversy surrounding mercury amalgam fillings, or are uncertain about how destructive they can be to your health, then sit down and relax, turn the page, and start reading. This book will change your life!

Tom McGuire, DDS
August 3, 2004

INTRODUCTION

The Hatter was the first to break the silence.
"What day of the month is it?" he said, turning to Alice:
he had taken his watch out of his pocket and was looking
at it uneasily shaking it every now and then, and hold-
ing it to his ear.
Alice considered a little, and then said "The fourth."
"Two days wrong!" sighed the Hatter.
"I told you butter wouldn't suit the works!" he added,
looking angrily at the March Hare....
"Some crumbs have got in as well," the Hatter grumbled:
"You shouldn't have put it in with the bread knife."
—Lewis Carroll, 1832-1898
From *Alice's Adventures in Wonderland*

Penned almost two centuries ago, Lewis Carroll's children's classic, *Alice's Adventures in Wonderland*, portrays a colorful fictional character who exhibits a quaint but somewhat erratic behavior—he is, after all, not altogether there. In creating his Mad Hatter, Carroll borrowed from the phrase "Mad as a Hatter," an 18th century expression that characterized the effects of chronic mercury exposure endured by those employed in the felt hat industry. Mad Hatter's disease, and the bizarre behavior of its victims, documents the long ago recognized effects of mercury toxicity.

According to the World Health Organization (WHO), there is no known safe level of mercury for humans. It is toxic in extraordinarily small amounts and each atom of mercury that enters the body will inflict harm. Mercury can damage every enzyme system and every structure in every cell of the body. Its most profound effect, however, is visited upon the central nervous system, the tissues in the brain and spinal chord.

Today, we know that mercury is the most toxic nonradioactive heavy metal on the planet—many times more poisonous than arsenic, lead, or cadmium. The tiniest amount of mercury, once absorbed by the body, can inflict widespread damage to cells, tissues and organs. Carried by the blood to the cells of the body, mercury:

- kills healthy cells;[1-3]

- penetrates and damages the blood-brain barrier[4] and accumulates in the motor function areas of the brain and central nervous system (CNS);[5-7]

- damages brain cells and nerve cells,[8] and generates high levels of reactive oxygen species (free radicals);[9,10]

- inhibits production of neurotransmitters, the chemical messengers of the nervous system;[11,12]

- disrupts the endocrine system, including the pituitary, adrenal, thyroid and thymus glands;[13-15]

- causes kidney malfunction;[16]

- is a reproductive and developmental toxin that severely impairs the ability to transport oxygen and nutrients to the fetus;[17,18]

- disrupts proper development of the brain;[19]

- causes learning disabilities and impairment, and a reduction in IQ;[20,21]

- increases the risks of cardiovascular disease and heart attack;[22,23]

- damages the immune system, resulting in several autoimmune disorders;[24]

- increases susceptibility to bacterial, viral, and fungal infections;[25-27] and

- causes significant destruction of stomach and intestinal epithelial cells.[28]

Mercury has been used by many cultures for thousands of years. The liquid metal and its derivatives have been found in Egyptian tombs dating back to 1500 B.C. As early as 2500 years ago some cultures were mixing it with other metals to form amalgams. The Romans used mercury in cosmetics to lighten the skin; the Greeks employed it to treat skin disorders, and the Chinese used cinnabar and calomel, the sulfide and chloride salts of mercury, in numerous medicinal remedies. For centuries, Europeans included mercury as an essential component of several medicines, including diuretics, antiseptics and laxatives, and in the late 1700s the metal became an essential ingredient in antisyphilitic agents because of its bactericidal effect. Mercury's efficacy is derived from the metal's profound and indiscriminating cytotoxicity—it kills cells with a vengeance.

It was during the 17th and 18th centuries that the dark side of mercury became evident, a consequence of its large-scale use in both medicine and manufacturing. In 1889, Charcot's *Clinical Lectures on Diseases of the Nervous System* attributed some types of rapid oscillatory tremors to mercury exposure. Later, environmental mercury exposure was identified with several cognitive impairments and behavioral disorders.

During the 1940s and 50s, mercury became synonymous with Pink Disease (acrodynia), caused by the use of teething powder and other baby products containing derivatives of mercury. The symptoms included a weepy red rash, peeling skin, lethargy, anemia, sensitivity to light, respiratory distress, and general ill health. About 25 percent of infants who contracted Pink Disease died.

In 1961, researchers in Japan linked elevated levels of mercury in the urine with the appearance of the mysterious Minamata disease. For some time, the affliction had plagued the residents of Minamata Bay with tremors, sensory loss, ataxia, and visual field constriction. Victims were diagnosed as having degeneration of their nervous systems, with numbness in limbs and lips, slurred speech, and constricted vision. Some suffered from involuntary movements; others lapsed into unconsciousness or suffered serious brain damage. Many were thought to be crazy when they began to shout uncontrollably.

The world awoke to the very real dangers of environmental mercury toxicity when it was finally revealed that a Japanese petrochemical manufacturer, rather than implement costly environmental control measures, had quietly dumped 27 tons of mercury compounds into Minamata Bay.

Following the Minamata disaster, industrial demand for mercury fell precipitously, largely as a result of aggressive federal bans on the use of the metal in paint and pesticides and the reduction of mercury in batteries.[29] In Canada, Europe and elsewhere, governments also took aggressive action to limit exposure to mercury compounds, as the effects of environmental contamination with this potent neurotoxin became increasingly clear.

Despite its notorious toxicity, mercury is still used in manufacturing, including the production of batteries, thermometers, barometers, semiconductors, electronic instruments, lighting, and chemicals. In addition, it is used in several industrial applications, such as electrical and power production, mining, electroplating, and jewelry making. The metal is also found in fungicides employed by the agricultural industry and in antiseptic agents and vaccine preservatives used in modern medicine.

Ironically, despite what we know about the toxic effects of mercury and despite the aggressive environmental control measures initiated to limit its use, one of the largest repositories of mercury today—and by far the greatest source of human exposure to this powerful neurological poison—are the thousands of tons of dental amalgams in the mouths of hundreds of millions of people, worldwide. Approximately 72 tons of mercury are placed in the mouths of North Americans every year—without *any* proof of safety.

An investigation of how this came to be, what it means to the health of millions of people of all ages—including those yet to be born—and what we can do about it, is why I have written this book.

CHAPTER 1

The History of the Mercury Amalgam Wars

"The absence of evidence is not evidence of absence."
—Dr. Carl Sagan, 1934-1996

Most people know there is a controversy surrounding amalgam fillings, but few are aware of the details. If you make inquiries about the issue of mercury poisoning through your dentist, it is unlikely you will receive much enlightenment. It is much more likely that you will be misled:

- If you should ask, "Is mercury poisonous?" your dentist will likely recite the standard response, dictated by the American Dental Association (ADA): "Not when used in dental amalgam ... when mercury is combined with other metals, such as silver, tin, and copper, it reacts with them to become a biologically inactive substance."[1]

- If you should ask, "Does mercury come out of my fillings if I eat or chew gum?" your dentist will likely reply, "Recent advances in both equipment and measurement techniques have allowed researchers to detect extremely low levels of mercury in patients' breath after they have chewed...but no evidence exists that associates this minute amount of mercury vapor with any toxic effects."[2]

- If you should ask, "Wouldn't it be wise for concerned patients to simply have their amalgam fillings removed and replaced with other materials?" your dentist will likely respond, "Unless a patient suffers an immediate adverse (allergic) reaction to an amalgam...it is not advisable to have amalgam fillings removed."[3]

All three of these position statements, promoted by the American (ADA) and Canadian (CDA) Dental Associations (the professional associations for dentistry in the United States and Canada), mislead the public and do not provide the information necessary for a patient to make an informed choice.

- On the first count, it is a fallacy that mercury is neutralized when it is combined with other components of dental amalgam. Mercury is merely diluted by the other components in what is essentially a "dynamic" solid. The toxin is still released as elemental mercury and, even in extremely small amounts, has profoundly toxic effects.[4-6]

- On the second count, the ADA/CDA response fails to recognize published experimental evidence dating back to 1926, indicating that mercury *is* released from amalgam fillings.[7] Researchers have more recently revealed intraoral mercury levels 30 to 100 times higher than the U.S. Environmental Protection Agency's (EPA) maximum allowable concentration for air that is safe for us to breathe.

- On the third count, the ADA position is based on its estimate of hypersensitivity to mercury of less than one percent of the population. This position is in stark contrast to the published scientific literature, which reports that allergies to mercury occur in approximately five percent of the population. Studies of those with amalgam fillings suggest that up to 35 percent develop hypersensitivity to mercury.[8]

Telling the story behind the controversy helps to explain why the dental industry has taken such a seemingly illogical and indefensible position regarding the use of mercury amalgam. To do this, we have to review the past 200 years of dental history.

Of Quicksilver and Quacks

In 1803, Joseph Fox, a prominent English dentist, invented a "fusible metal" filling that, when placed in a cavity in molten form and allowed to cool, would solidify to the exact shape of the cavity. Later, August Taveau of Paris and Thomas Bell of England both conceived the idea of mixing shavings from silver coins with mercury to create an amalgam filling material that would be soft during insertion but harden very quickly. In 1833, the use of mercury amalgam was introduced to the United States by the Crawcour brothers, two French entrepreneurs who made extravagant claims for this new material. They called it *Royal Mineral Succedaneum* because the amalgam was supposed to take the place of the royal mineral, gold.

Compared to what had previously been used to fill teeth, such as molten lead, pine resin, stone, woodchips, cork, tin foil, and gold foil, mercury amalgam was revolutionary. The filling material was relatively inexpensive, placement could be completed in one visit, and it lasted a relatively long time. Soon, amalgam fillings became the rage. They were at once desirable and affordable, and dentists benefited because the new filling material created a greater demand for their services—along with, of course, more profit.

It did not take long, however, for controversy regarding the safety of mercury amalgams to arise. Scientists and medical professionals were already well aware that mercury was poisonous and that these mercury-containing fillings might pose a significant health hazard. Many early dentists expressed similar concerns about possible mercury poisoning, as it was widely recognized that mercury exposure resulted in many overt reactions, including dementia and a loss of motor skills. Once these

It is interesting to note that the German term for mercury is "quecksilber" and the German pronunciation for queck is "quack." For this reason, dentists who placed mercury amalgams, at that time, came to be known as "quacks." The term has now come to mean anyone who is an "ignorant pretender of medical skill."

concerns about toxicity came to the forefront, amalgam use was soon denounced by the medical profession as well as by a substantial number of dentists.

AMALGAM WAR I

In the United States during the early 1800s, there were two types of dentists: medical dentists and barber dentists. Medical dentists were physicians who also practiced dentistry; barber dentists were people involved in various non-medical trades, such as barbering, blacksmithing and carpentering—or anyone else who thought working on teeth might be profitable. During this period there were no dental schools, no dental associations, and no laws that prevented anyone from hanging a shingle on their door to offer dental services.

Concern about mercury toxicity provoked the medical dentists to prevent the barber dentists from indiscriminately exposing the public to what was clearly a poison. Realizing that the barber dentists would not stop using amalgams, the medical dentists established the first U.S. dental school. In 1840, they also established the first national dental association, calling it the American Society of Dental Surgeons (ASDS). In 1843, the ASDS took up the cause of banning the use of dental amalgams, and the ensuing controversy erupted into what dental historians call the Amalgam Wars.

> *In 1848, the ASDS found eleven of its New York members guilty of malpractice for using mercury amalgams and suspended them.*

The Society's approach was to standardize the practice of dentistry, much like the medical profession, by establishing specific rules and regulations and a governing body with the clout to enforce them. The purpose was to prevent all non-medical dentists from the practice of dentistry and to prohibit further use of mercury amalgam. In 1843, once it had consolidated power, the ASDS passed a resolution banning the use of amalgam fillings by any licensed dentist. The ASDS resolution declared that the use of amalgam fillings constituted malpractice and those who continued to use the substance could lose their license to practice dentistry. In 1848, the Society found eleven of its New York members guilty of malpractice for using mercury amalgams and subsequently suspended them.

> *The ASDS resolution declared that the use of amalgam fillings constituted malpractice and those who continued to use the substance could lose their license to practice dentistry.*

Unfortunately, the ASDS resolution, while mandatory within its own membership, was not legally binding. What could influence ASDS members did nothing to stop the barber dentists who were not part of the Society—and who cared little about the health hazards of mercury—from using amalgams. Nor, as it turned out, did the resolution stop an increasing number of ASDS members, who were more concerned about maximizing profit than protecting patients' health.

Over the next 16 years, an ever-growing number of ASDS dentists saw countless patients lost to barber dentists. They realized that if they were not able to use the easy-to-insert and inexpensive amalgam, they would continue to lose business. Seeing this, a number of ASDS dentists conspired to form their own dental association.

In a cunning tactical maneuver, the rogue members absented themselves from the Annual General Meeting of the Society, August 1st, 1856, and the organization was subsequently dissolved for lack of a quorum. No longer were dental practitioners bound by the ASDS antiamalgam resolution. Former ASDS members were now free to place as many amalgam fillings as they could find teeth in which to cram them—and *without* the threat of losing their license to practice.

> *Today, an ADA member dentist who removes an amalgam filling for health reasons can lose his license to practice dentistry.*

In 1859, following the demise of the ASDS, representatives of several state dental societies met in Niagara Falls, New York, and formed a new national organization, the American Dental Association (ADA). Thus was born the regulatory body that continues to control the U.S. dental profession today. Under this new authority, the regulations governing the use of amalgams were the antithesis of the rules of the original ASDS.

Ironically, while it was the medical dentists who recognized mercury as a health hazard, and it was the medical profession that declared it unethical to use mercury fillings, it was the non-medical barber dentists who held the winning hand. This was the issue upon which the practice of dentistry and the practice of medicine parted ways. In essence, the fracturing of dentistry from medicine occurred over a medical health issue, not a dental one; tragically, the fundamental reason for the split was not to improve the practice of dentistry or to provide better treatment to the patient, but for the pursuit of profit.

The first stage of the Amalgam Wars had proved victorious for the conventional forces. Despite the growing scientific evidence demonstrating the toxicity of dental amalgams, the scientists, medical practitioners and informed public of the antiamalgam faction had been forced, for the time being, to concede defeat.

PAPERING OVER THE FACTS

The answer to the question, "Why would a health professional knowingly put mercury into anyone's mouth?" created a problem for the newly formed ADA. They knew they could never argue that mercury was safe—even in the 1840s every physician and scientist knew that mercury was a powerful poison. Aware that the scientific and medical professions would continue to be formidable adversaries, the members of the newly formed association understood that they would have a difficult time defending their use of mercury. The public simply would not accept the concept of filling anyone's mouth with a poison. Clearly, the ADA had to find another way to put an end to the escalating dispute.

The solution was to declare the issue of toxicity a moot point. Honing the argument that once mercury is mixed with other metals it reacts to form a biologically inactive substance, the ADA declared that mercury simply is not released from the amalgam and, consequently, the toxic effect is eliminated. End of story.

To the ADA this was also the end of the battle and, astoundingly, the Association has used this argument to defend its position for the past 160 years. While the ADA's declaration did force a temporary retreat, it certainly did not end the war.

During the past 160 years, scientists, health professionals, antiamalgam groups, and a small but increasingly vocal group of dentists have consistently challenged the ADA's position regarding the safety of amalgam fillings. Unfortunately, for most of those years the technology was not available to verify that mercury was, indeed, released from amalgam. On the other hand, the ADA could not prove that mercury was not released, nor did it ever make any attempt to do so. The ADA, instead, relied on its political clout to silence the guns of the antiamalgam forces.

Nonetheless, the antiamalgam faction simply refused to accept the ADA's denials. They knew, from the basic laws of solution chemistry, that mercury must be released from amalgam fillings. Invoking the Hippocratic doctrine of "First, do no harm," the antiamalgam forces took the position that, until the safety of mercury amalgam could be demonstrated conclusively, it should not be placed in anyone's teeth. While lacking the hard scientific evidence that would sway the ADA, the antiamalgam forces felt they had an abundance of anecdotal evidence to support their position. For proof, they turned to patients who had amalgams in their teeth. The evidence revealed that a high percentage of patients with a wide range of mercury-related symptoms improved significantly after their amalgam fillings were removed.

While this impressed the dentists who removed the fillings and the patients whose health improved, it certainly did not influence the ADA, which discounted the anecdotal evidence as "unscientific." The ADA had a valid point and it rested on the need for rigorous scientific verification— a technological quandary that would confound the antiamalgam forces until German researchers finally confirmed that mercury is released in measurable amounts from amalgam fillings.[9] This long-awaited scientific proof set the stage for the second phase of the amalgam wars.

Amalgam War II

The Second Amalgam War was initiated in the 1920s, when Professor Alfred Stock, a chemist at the Kaiser Wilhelm Institute in Germany, published research in leading journals of the day demonstrating significant adverse effects from amalgam fillings. While the evidence was compelling and the resulting debate intense, the dispute faded away when the storm of the real World War II erupted on the national stage.

It was not until 1957 that researchers, using a radioactive mercury tracer, showed that placement of amalgam fillings in both humans and dogs resulted in significant elevations of mercury in the urine and feces.[10] This finding was followed by a number of clinical studies confirming that mercury vapor released in the mouth led to an increased uptake of mercury in body tissues.[11-17] Most damaging to the ADA claim that mercury in amalgams is not released, Canadian researchers, in 1985, showed that mercury vapor increased dramatically when the amalgam was stimulated by chewing. These findings have been documented by numerous subsequent studies, all of which confirm a startling increase in mercury vapor as a consequence of any activity which stimulates the amalgam.

Nonetheless, the ADA continued to remain resolute in its defense of the indefensible. While quietly admitting that amalgam fillings do, indeed, release mercury, the Association now refused to recognize that the *amount* of mercury released is unsafe. While grudgingly letting go of one controversy, the ADA was quick to create another.

Amalgam War III

Modern methods of detecting mercury vapor, introduced in the 1970s, paved the way for the Third Amalgam War, which was ignited in 1985. The International Academy of Oral Medicine and Toxicology (IAOMT), a Canadian-based organization dedicated to research and education in oral health issues, reviewed the findings of the National Institute of Dental Research (NIDR) on the biocompatibility of metals in dentistry.[18] Based on the available literature of the day, the Academy concluded that there was substantial doubt about the safety of amalgam fillings and recommended a moratorium on the use of mercury amalgams.

The battle heated up considerably with a 1989 ruling by the U.S. Environmental Protection Agency (EPA), which classified mercury amalgam as a hazardous substance. This was followed by a blistering exposé on the safety of mercury amalgam by the CBS television program, *60 Minutes*, aired in 1990. The resulting public outcry led to a U.S. Food and Drug Administration (FDA) hearing, a conference sponsored by NIDR, and a call for a review of the scientific literature by the U.S Public Health Service.

The ADA, furious over the bad publicity it was receiving, went on the offensive, claiming the scientific evidence showed that amalgam fillings were safe. Dentists all over the country received a blizzard of ADA information circulars; two-minute "news" videos heralding the safety of amalgam fillings were distributed to television stations across the land. In Canada, the Canadian Dental Association (CDA) also raised the flag, joining the charge with its U.S. counterpart, the ADA. Adhering to the maxim of, "when the facts are with you, pound the facts and when the facts are against you, pound the table," the ADA pounded the table. Muskets leveled—but with no ammunition in the breach—the ADA's offensive proved hollow. These announcements failed to offer a scintilla of credible scientific evidence supporting their position.

In April, 1990, the ADA also published a special report, which was circulated to dental practitioners throughout the country. The report, *When your Patients Ask about Mercury in Amalgam*,[19] presented a number of questions and answers clearly designed to assuage the public concern about amalgam fillings. According to the IAOMT, the ADA special report was a misleading fabrication that contained sufficient misinformation to cause serious consequences and prevent patients from making an informed decision—leaving the dental practitioner at risk of liability and negligent misrepresentation.[20]

In its response to the ADA *Special Report*, the IAOMT refuted all of the association's claims regarding the safety of amalgams and presented hard scientific evidence to back its statements. The IAOMT castigated the ADA for its failure to provide any scientific evidence to the contrary. The Academy further charged that that the association had been remiss in not protecting the public and members of the dental profession from personal harm due to exposure to mercury amalgams.[21]

A MOUTHFUL OF POISON

In 1991, Dr. Boyd Haley, of the University of Kentucky, uncovered impressive evidence of mercury amalgam toxicity while studying Alzheimer's disease. Haley's examination of Alzheimer's-affected brain cells suggested to him that there had to be a toxicant—a toxic substance that caused the disease. He later identified two environmental sources that could be culprits: cadmium (found mainly in cigarette smoke) and mercury.

Aware that dental amalgams had been found to leak mercury into the body, Haley devised a controlled experiment, placing dental amalgam and healthy brain tissue in the same medium. He observed that only a few weeks' exposure of the brain tissue to mercury amalgam was sufficient to markedly suppress the secretion of tubulin, an important enzyme that regulates critical brain functions. His findings were consistent with the effects observed in mercury toxicity and with brain tissue affected by Alzheimer's disease. Haley's experiment conclusively demonstrated two important points:

- there is demonstrable release of mercury from amalgam fillings; and

- there is a significant and harmful effect of mercury on brain tissue that is consistent with that observed in Alzheimer's disease.

According to Haley, the release of mercury from amalgams likely exposed those with amalgam fillings to chronic low-dose mercury leakage.[22] Haley's conclusions are backed by numerous recent studies that point the finger at mercury amalgam as the primary source of chronic mercury poisoning.[23,24]

Recent studies in animals and humans also confirm the presence of mercury from amalgam fillings in tissues, amniotic fluid and urine.[25-27] Moreover, it appears that childhood learning difficulties, and even autism, may be primarily the result of mercury poisoning. Autism, virtually unknown before World War II, has become widespread in North America. Its prevalence corresponds to the increased use of mercury during this period.[28]

Commenting on the organized resistance of the dental profession, Dr. Jordan Davis, co-director of the Toxic Studies Institute of Boca Raton,

Florida, reflects, "There has been [resistance] for a very long time because they have a lot to lose. Dentists have pride, reputation, money, and liability on the line. To admit that they have mistakenly been using a harmful substance to treat tooth decay for many years is a very difficult confession to make—and it is fraught with extremely serious consequences."[29]

The ADA now argues before the United States' courts that it bears no culpability for its position with regard to amalgam fillings. Indeed, the same organization that has invested so much in becoming the perceived authority over the practice of dentistry, both to the profession *and to the public*, now suggests that it, incredibly, bears no legal responsibility for the advice it gives. It appears that dental practitioners, and the public, who have faithfully followed the ADA mantra may well have been hung out to dry by the association they have come to trust.

> *"One of these days there's going to be a mammoth lawsuit about mercury fillings similar to one that's already been filed in Canada. It's going to be bigger than what we've seen over tobacco. It's going to hit people like a Mack truck that putting mercury in their teeth amounts to putting poison in their mouths. Once they realize that in no uncertain terms, they're going to be angry."*
>
> —Dr. Charles Williamson,
> Toxic Studies Institute

CHAPTER 2

Mercury, Mercury Everywhere

When Jove sent blessings to all men that are,
And Mercury conveyed them in a jar,
That friend of tricksters introduced by stealth
Disease for the apothecary's health,
Whose gratitude impelled him to proclaim:
"My deadliest drug shall bear my patron's name!"
— Ambrose Bierce (1842-1914)
The Devil's Dictionary

There is considerable release of elemental mercury into the atmosphere and into our inland and coastal waters as a consequence of natural processes and modern industrial activity. While most nations are now implanting stringent control measures to reduce mercury contamination, there remains substantial room for improvement. Mercury in our environment is, indeed, a growing threat. But, how does it compare to the mercury in our mouths?

ATMOSPHERIC

Mercury vapor is dispersed across the globe by prevailing winds, where it has an atmospheric residence of up to three years, returning to the earth through rainfall and accumulating in the soil and water.

Major atmospheric sources of mercury include degassing of the earth's crust, volcanic activity, and evaporation from natural bodies of water. These sources contribute approximately 2,970 to 6,600 tons per year. Industrial emissions, however, add considerably to this annual output. The total global atmospheric release of mercury, due to human activities, exceeds 3,300 tons per year (1990).[1]

In 1994, electricity generated with fossil fuels was responsible for 23 percent of all industrial atmospheric mercury emissions, with coal-fired power plants producing the most mercury. Living downwind from any facility that releases mercury into the environment will expose you to mercury in the air. Consequently, the surrounding area will also have greater soil, river, lake, and groundwater contamination.

Data for the estimated atmospheric release of mercury in the United Kingdom (1985) shows that the burning of fossil fuels contributed the greatest amount—some 25,500 kilograms per year—followed by:

- the production and use of products and materials containing mercury;
- municipal waste incineration;
- nonferrous metal production;
- cement manufacturing;
- steel production; and
- sewage sludge incineration.[2,3]

In developing countries, the emissions from industry and mining are probably much greater.

Soil- and Water-borne

Once deposited in the water and soil through rainfall, elemental and inorganic mercury is converted to methylmercury through microbial action. Methylmercury, a highly toxic substance, then enters aquatic and terrestrial food chains through uptake by organisms and plants. Mercury binds tightly to plant proteins, the first step in the bioaccumulation of this powerful toxin. This is followed by consumption of the plant tissue by herbivores and subsequent predation by higher life forms.

As the toxin ascends the food chain, biomagnification (increasing concentration in the tissues of predators) occurs, attaining its highest levels in those predatory species at the top of the food chain. The level of methylmercury in the tissues of aquatic species can reach 10,000 to 100,000 times the concentration in the water. Levels exceeding 1.2 mg/kg are often found in Mediterranean tuna, swordfish, mackerel and shark. Similar levels have been observed in freshwater species, such as trout, pike, walleye and bass, taken from polluted lakes and rivers.

In Canada and Sweden, there has been a marked increase in methylmercury concentration in aquatic life following the construction of dams and reservoirs.[4] Because of its extreme toxicity, one-half gram of mercury will contaminate an entire ten acre lake to the extent that a health warning and a ban on consumption of fish is required. Throughout the U.S., over 50,000 lakes and seven percent of all river systems post warnings that either ban or limit consumption of fish, due to unacceptable levels of mercury. In both Canada and the U.S., all the Great Lakes and many coastal bays and estuaries carry similar health warnings.[5]

INDUSTRIAL

In the early 1990s, worldwide mining of mercury yielded about 11,000 tons of the metal per year. These activities release additional mercury into the environment through atmospheric discharge and the dumping of mine tailings.[6]

Other important sources of mercury include the combustion of fossil fuels, the smelting of metal ores, the refining of gold and production of cement, refuse incineration, and the industrial applications of metals.

There are over 3,000 industrial uses for mercury and its various compounds. Table 2-1, while not exhaustive, includes the more common industrial uses of mercury. If you do not know if your employer uses mercury, check with the appropriate department. If you suspect that a product you use may contain mercury, write to the company and ask. Workers who manufacture products containing mercury and those who purchase these products are risking avoidable exposure to this harmful environmental toxin. Fortunately, mercury is now gradually being eliminated from many food and personal-use products.

Table 2-1

Industrial Uses of Mercury

Acetaldehyde Production	Germicidal Agents
Antiseptics	Histology Products
Antisyphilitic Agents	Ink Manufacturing
Bactericides	Infrared Detectors
Barometers	Insecticidal Products
Batteries	Manometers
Bronzing	Mercury Amalgam Fillings
Calibration Devices	Metal Mining and Production
Chemical Laboratories	Mirror Silvering
Chlor-alkali Production	Mercury and Neon Lamps
Cosmetics	Paints
Diaper Products	Paper Pulp Products
Electric Switches	Pathology Reagents
Electroplating	Perfumes
Embalming Agents	Photography Reagents
Explosives	Polyurethane Foam Production
Fabric Softeners	Seed Preservation
Farming Industry	Semi-Conductor Cells
Finger Printing Products	Spermicidal Jellies
Floor Wax and Polish	Tattooing Inks
Fluorescent Lamps	Taxidermy
Fossil Fuel Production/Combustion	Thermometers
Fungicidal Products	Vaccine Preservatives
Fur Hat Processing	Wood Preservatives

DENTAL

Although tougher laws are being enacted in many countries, mercury
released from dental offices remains a significant source of environmental
contamination. Data from a 1976 World Health Organization
(WHO) report indicate that, in industrialized countries at that time,

approximately three percent of the total consumption of mercury was used for dental amalgam.[7] The compound is used for 75 to 80 percent of all tooth restorations, and in the U.S. it is estimated that every dentist uses between 0.9 to 1.4 kg (2.0 to 3.1 pounds) of amalgam per year.

In Chapter 4 we will review the various regulatory agencies and the guidelines they have established to protect the public health. Considering that the ADA is the largest professional organization of dental practitioners in the U.S., a vocation heavily involved with mercury in the workplace, it is remarkable that the association has never established its own guidelines or monitoring protocols for mercury exposure.

Advances in both equipment and measurement techniques have allowed researchers to determine intraoral mercury levels in dental patients that are 30 to 100 times higher than the Environmental Protection Agency's maximum allowable concentration for air quality (set at 0.3 parts per million).[8-11] Despite this, the ADA has not implemented a program for patient/practitioner monitoring, nor does it acknowledge the dangers posed by mercury amalgams and the need for the establishment of procedures involved in their removal and replacement. At first, the ADA's position seems absurd—until you consider that, to do so, the ADA would need to establish a "safe" level of exposure that would be dramatically higher than those levels established by other regulatory agencies. Otherwise, patients would have to leave the dental office, as their mouths would constitute a hazardous worksite for dental staff!

This point is brought home poignantly by Dr. Tano Lucero, former research chemist and industrial hygienist for the U.S. Occupational Safety and Health Administration (OSHA). Dr. Lucero had become a victim of neurotoxic poisoning related to his job. Following advice that he should have his amalgams removed, he discovered that his intraoral mercury levels were almost twice the OSHA standard of 50 $\mu g/m^3$ per 8-hour shift, but he was being exposed to this level for 24 hours a day. Says Lucero, "If I were doing an OSHA inspection of my mouth, I would be in violation of the OSHA standard and subject to serious citation, which carries a $1,000 penalty!"[12]

RELATIVE HUMAN EXPOSURES

Considering the many avenues for environmental and occupational exposure to mercury, including exposure through contaminated food sources, people with amalgam fillings are particularly vulnerable to toxic overload of mercury. Working in a business that uses mercury, using products that contain mercury, and living near facilities that release mercury into the air, water, and soil, dramatically increase the risk of taking in more mercury than government regulations allow, even among those who don't have amalgam fillings.

In 1990, the WHO estimated the amount of mercury intake from a variety of sources. The following table shows the average daily intake and retention of total mercury and mercury compounds in the general population not occupationally exposed to mercury.

Table 2-2

Estimated Daily Intake & Retention of Mercury

Source	Type	Av. Daily Intake µg/day	Av. Daily Retention µg/day
Amalgam Fillings	Elemental Mercury	3.8 - 21	3 - 17
Fish	Methyl/Inorganic Mercury	3.0	2.3
Other Food	Inorganic Mercury	3.6	0.25
Air	All types	0.04	0.031
Water	All types	0.05	0.0035
TOTAL		10.6 - 27.7 µg/day	5.58 - 19.6 µg/day

Adapted from Environmental Health Criteria 101: Methylmercury (WHO, 1990)[13]

According to the WHO data, mercury released from amalgam fillings is, by wide measure, the primary source of exposure. With an estimated average daily intake ranging from 3.8 to 21 micrograms (µg) per day, exposure from amalgams is between 6 to 7 times the intake from fish or other food sources and 400 to 500 times the level of environmental intake.

However, it is still important to keep in mind that, while amalgam fillings are certainly number one on the hit list, they are not the only source of exposure. For this reason, one cannot evaluate in isolation the harm that amalgam fillings may be doing to your health. All sources of mercury exposure must be considered—including that from thimerosal, a mercury-based preservative used in vaccines, which was not considered in the WHO report.

In summary, millions of people are exposed to mercury through their workplace, their environment, the products they use, and their diet. However, while the amount of mercury absorbed from exposure to various environmental and occupational sources can be substantial, it pales when compared to the amount of mercury absorbed from amalgam fillings. Simply put, if you are walking around with mercury in your mouth, you are your own primary exposure risk to mercury—and you will have to live with it every day until you do something about it.

CHAPTER 3

The Poisonous Nature of Mercury

"Mercury vapor is toxic—period."
— Dr. Charles Williamson,
Toxic Studies Institute

Mercury is the only metal that is liquid in its elemental state. Its chemical symbol, Hg, is derived from the Greek word *hydrargyrias*, meaning water silver. At room temperature, the liquid metal releases vapor as a poisonous, odorless and colorless gas. The amount released increases with temperature. Once inhaled, mercury vapor readily passes from the lungs and immediately enters the bloodstream. What is not stored in the blood cells quickly diffuses into the cells and tissues throughout the body. The fact that elemental mercury, the same form used in amalgam fillings, releases mercury vapor at room temperature, explains why the metal is so much more poisonous than other heavy metals.

There are three forms of mercury: elemental, inorganic and organic. While all forms of mercury are extremely poisonous, organic mercury is by far the most toxic, followed by the elemental and then the inorganic forms of the metal.

Elemental mercury is not chemically bonded with other elements; it is mercury in its purest form. It vaporizes easily and is quickly absorbed into the body through inhalation. Elemental mercury passes through the bloodstream and accumulates in fatty tissues, such as the brain. It crosses the blood-brain barrier, where it becomes ionized and subsequently trapped. The elemental mercury that is inhaled is converted to an inorganic ionic form, which also becomes trapped behind the blood-brain barrier, contributing to its powerful toxic effect.[1] Elemental mercury can also cross the placental barrier to accumulate in the fetus.

Inorganic mercury is mercury that is chemically bonded with inorganic elements to form mercurous and mercuric salts. One example is cinnabar, the red sulfide of mercury that was mined by the Romans for its mercury content and has been the main commercial source of mercury throughout the centuries. Inorganic mercury is absorbed orally or transdermally (through the skin). While low in fat solubility, inorganic mercury is extremely toxic, damages the kidneys, and is slow to be eliminated from the body.[2]

Organic mercury includes the carbon-containing compounds of mercury, such as methyl mercury, the most prevalent form found in environmental contamination. Organic mercurials are absorbed more completely by the gastrointestinal tract than are inorganic mercury salts. Once absorbed, most of the organic mercurials are converted into their inorganic forms and possess toxicities similar to inorganic mercury. Like elemental mercury, organic mercurials are highly fat soluble and consequently are distributed throughout the body, accumulating in the brain, liver, kidneys, hair and skin. Organic mercury also crosses the placental barrier to accumulate in the fetus.

A PERVASIVE TOXICITY

A particularly challenging characteristic of mercury is its ubiquitous toxicity. The metal can poison every enzyme, damage every cellular structure, and kill virtually every cell in the body. This explains the extraordinary diversity of symptoms and diseases that are directly and indirectly attributed to mercury poisoning. Mercuric toxins can also seriously deplete essential minerals, including zinc, magnesium, and copper. No matter where mercury is in the body, it is harmful for as long as it is present.

Most of the symptoms related to mercury toxicity are neurological. Mercury is primarily recognized as a neurotoxin because it has its most profound effect on the central nervous system (CNS). The neurons of the

CNS are composed mostly of fats and, as previously mentioned, both elemental and organic mercury are highly fat-soluble. Consequently, elemental and organic mercury have a high affinity for nerve cells and readily cross the blood-brain barrier, which is the protective vascular membrane that separates the brain from the rest of the body. Once inside the brain, these forms of mercury have a particularly destructive effect on the nerve cells. After reacting with and damaging neurons, the mercury is oxidized and converted to a less soluble inorganic form that becomes trapped within the brain.

PERSISTENCE IN THE BODY

The term *biological half-life* refers to the time it takes to remove one-half of the amount of a substance from the body. The biological half-life of a substance can vary, depending on its location in the body. While the half-life of inorganic mercury in the kidneys and other body tissues can be as brief as 64 days, it is estimated that the half-life of inorganic mercury in the brain is in excess of 20 years.[3] This means that in 20 years, half the mercury that was there initially would still be there. In another 20 years, one-half of that half will still be there, and so on.

Even if you eliminate all sources of mercury exposure (including the removal of all dental amalgams) but do nothing to support your body's ability to remove the accumulated mercury, it will take years—perhaps a lifetime—for your body to eliminate this poison. Mercury will not just disappear on its own, and if your body is not able to eliminate it, the poison will stay in your body forever. The fact is, mercury is removed atom by atom through the actions of the body's detoxification systems, including several powerful antioxidants (substances manufactured by our cells or supplied through our diet that reduce oxidative damage). Antioxidants can chelate (bind) with the poison to remove it from the cells and carry it out of the body. However, if your body is deficient in antioxidants or the detoxification systems of your cells are impaired—or if there is simply too much mercury entering your body—this elimination process can be overwhelmed. While it may be years before observable symptoms become evident, mercury will continue to accumulate and will quietly, but inexorably, exact its toll on your health.

Fortunately, if the sources of mercury contamination are removed and our bodies' detoxification systems are given optimal nutritional support,

the process of mercury detoxification can be markedly accelerated. Ways
to do this will be discussed in detail in a later chapter of this book.

Symptoms

Mercury poisoning can result in serious pathological challenges, including:
renal failure, cardiovascular disturbances, dementia, neurological dysfunctions, liver and digestive disorders, immune dysfunctions, allergic
responses, hormonal imbalances, and learning disorders—to name but a
few. The elemental form of mercury can be converted in the body to its
more toxic form and can cause visual disturbances, ataxia, hearing loss,
general mental deterioration, and muscle tremors. With acute exposure,
organic mercury intoxication can lead to kidney failure, paralysis and death.

A potent neurotoxin, mercury targets the brain, including: the cerebral
cortex, motor and sensory centers, the temporal cortex (hearing), and the
cerebellum (muscle coordination). Evidence also suggests that cumulative
mercury toxicity may be added to the growing roster of maladies associated
with autoimmune disorders.[4] At least 100 symptoms are believed to be
directly or indirectly related to mercury poisoning; the number and
severity are dependent on a variety of factors. None of the symptoms of
chronic mercury poisoning are unique—other toxins and physiological
disturbances can mimic these symptoms and frustrate a positive diagnosis
of mercury toxicity.

The only way that anyone, including a health professional, can be certain
that mercury did not cause or contribute to a particular symptom is to
know definitively that the victim has not been exposed to mercury. For
example, mercury certainly is not the only thing that causes headaches;
however, chronic exposure to mercury can make headaches more fre-
quent and severe. Table 3-1 lists the numerous symptoms related to
chronic mercury toxicity.

Table 3-1

Common Symptoms of Chronic Mercury Poisoning

Emotions	Nose	Lungs
Aggressiveness	Inflammation	Asthma
Anger	Sinusitis	Bronchitis
Anxiety	Stuffy Nose	Chest Congestion
Confusion	Excessive Mucus Formation	Shortness of Breath
Depression		
Fear (Recurrent)	**Head**	**Other**
Hallucinations	Dizziness	Allergies
	Faintness	Anorexia
Muscles & Joints	Headaches (Recurrent)	Excessive Blushing
Cramping	Ringing In Ears	Genital Discharge
Joint Pain		Gland Swelling
Muscle Pain	**Digestive System**	Hair Loss
Weakness	Colitis	Illnesses (Recurrent)
	Loss of Appetite	Insomnia
Neurological & Mental	Weight Loss	Loss of Sense of Smell
Tremors	Nausea/Vomiting	Perspiration (Excessive)
Lack Of Concentration		Kidney Failure
Learning Disorders	**Energy Levels**	Skin (Cold and Clammy)
Memory Loss	Apathy	Skin Problems
Numbness	Chronic Fatigue	Vision Problems (Tunnel Vision)
Slurred Speech	Restlessness	Edema (Water Retention)

Oral/Throat	Heart
Bad Breath	Anemia
Burning Sensation	Chest Pain
Chronic Cough	Rapid or Irregular Heartbeat
Gingivitis/Bleeding Gums	
Leukoplakia (White Patches)	
Metallic Taste	
Sore Throat	
Ulcers of Oral Cavity	

DISEASES RELATED TO MERCURY POISONING

When it comes to establishing the causative link between mercury and disease, it is important to consider the numerous related risk factors that can produce similar symptoms. Each individual, depending on his or her particular lifestyle, nutritional status, and genetic and emotional makeup, will respond differently to cumulative mercury poisoning. One thing, however, is certain: the probability of developing a related health problem dramatically increases when related risk factors *and* mercury are present together.

The relationship between mercury poisoning, associated risk factors, and the severity and nature of disease symptoms has critical implications for medical diagnosis and treatment. For those patients who have amalgam fillings, health professionals should consider that chronic mercury poisoning will exacerbate virtually every disease symptom. Moreover, if both the source of mercury exposure and the accumulated mercury in the body are not removed, success in treating any disease will be compromised. Simply put, if you are currently suffering from any of the symptoms or diseases listed in this chapter, you must do everything possible to determine if mercury is a contributing factor. Otherwise, your body's efforts to heal itself will be futile.

Mercury exposure has been linked to the diseases listed in Table 3-2. New research, demonstrating the destructive effect of mercury toxicity on the immune system, promises to make the list much longer.[5-9]

Table 3-2

Diseases Related to Mercury Poisoning

Acrodynia	Emphysema
Alzheimer's	Fibromyalgia
Amyotrophic Lateral Sclerosis	Hormonal Dysfunction
Asthma	Intestinal Dysfunction
Arthritis	Immune System Disorders
Autism	Kidney Disease
Candida	Learning Disorders
Cardiovascular Disease	Liver Disorders
Crohn's Disease	Metabolic Encephalopathy
Chronic Fatique Syndrome	Multiple Sclerosis
Depression	Reproductive Disorders
Developmental Defects	Parkinson's
Diabetes	Senile Dementia
Eczema	Thyroid Disease

Diseases Related to Mercury Poisoning

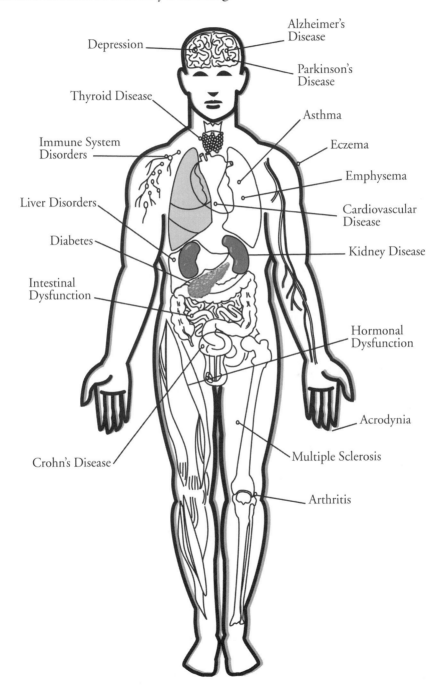

For those who have a mouthful of amalgam, you must understand that you will never be truly healthy as long as these fillings are releasing mercury into your body.

ALLERGY TO MERCURY—MAKING A BAD SITUATION WORSE

In a 1984 article in *Science Digest*, the American Dental Association estimated that five percent of the population is sensitive to mercury. This means that the number of people in the United States with mercury allergies could, at the time, have exceeded 7.5 million. Curiously, the ADA has subsequently, and unexplainably, revised its estimate downward to less than one percent, claiming that there have been only 100 documented cases of mercury allergy.

Fortunately, the ADA is not the only source of information about the percentage of people in the United States allergic to mercury. Other estimates range up to 35 percent,[10] providing as many as 103 million Americans who may be sensitive to mercury.

If you are allergic to mercury, you are dealing with a multifaceted problem: the direct and indirect effects of mercury poisoning as well as the effects of an allergic reaction that is atypical of other allergic responses. Generally speaking, an allergy occurs after exposure to an allergen in products, seasonal plants or particular foods. Once identified, most of these sources can be eliminated or removed with relative ease. For someone allergic to wheat, it is a simple thing to remove the grain from the diet. However, for someone allergic to mercury, you cannot remove the allergen unless you remove mercury from your workplace and environment, including the fillings in your teeth *and* the mercury that has accumulated in your body. Until such action is taken, you will be exposed to this allergen every minute of every day—what a burden on your immune system and your entire body!

Another important aspect of allergic reactions, which determines the severity of the reaction, is the extent of exposure. For example, you could be allergic to ragweed and have no adverse response if you breathe in only a few grains of the pollen. However, if someone shook the weed in your face, exposing you to millions of grains, you could have a serious adverse reaction.

Similarly, if you are allergic to mercury and are exposed to low levels in the workplace your allergic response could be tolerable, with low-grade symptoms that probably would not seriously affect your quality of life. However, if your occupation exposes you to material amounts of mercury, you have amalgam fillings and you engage in activities that stimulate your amalgams frequently, it is likely that your response to the mercury will be far greater and could overwhelm your immune system.

Most people have likely never considered their amalgam fillings as a possible cause or contributor to their allergies. It is just as unlikely that many individuals have ever been cautioned of this possibility by their dentist or health professional.

Signs and Symptoms of Mercury Allergy

Although testing is the best way to accurately diagnose an allergy to mercury, there are also a number of signs and symptoms to watch for. These signs and symptoms are elusive. They may result from exposure to a variety of sources, and a causal link to mercury poisoning can be

Table 3-3

Common Allergy Symptoms

Absentmindedness	Muscle Pain
Breathing Difficulties	Nasal Congestion
Burning Eyes	Nausea
Difficulties In Concentration	Nose Itchy, Runny, Or Tingling
Cough	Postnasal Drip
Depression	Pulse (Rapid)
Diarrhea	Smell Impairment
Dizziness	Skin Rashes Or Itch
Ear Ringing	Sleeping Difficulties
Eyes Watery, Itchy, Crusty, Or Red	Sneezing
Flushing	Swallowing (Difficult)
Headaches	Swelling
Heart Palpitations	Throat Irritation, Itching
Hives	Tiredness
Irritability	Vomiting
Joint Aches & Pains	Wheezing

identified only when you *knowingly* change your level of mercury exposure. A change in your work environment, your eating habits (such as if you begin consuming mercury-contaminated fish), or in the products you use are all opportunities for you to identify mercury-allergy based symptoms.

Indeed, if you have amalgam fillings implanted or removed, you should closely monitor any symptoms identified in the following table to see if any are associated with the change in your exposure level.

These are generalized indications of an allergy. They have special meaning in the context of mercury sensitivity if they appear or increase in severity during amalgam placement or removal. If you are unsure or curious about the source of your symptoms, consult with an allergy specialist. A good way to test for a mercury allergy is to use the MELISA® test, which measures hypersensitivity to metals, including mercury.

MELISA® research shows that any allergy to metals, including mercury, may aggravate the diseases shown in Table 3-4:

Table 3-4

Diseases Aggravated by Allergy to Metals

Amyotrophic Lateral Sclerosis	Multiple Chemical Sensitivity
Chronic Fatique Syndrome	Multiple Sclerosis
Crohn's Disease	Myalgic Encephalitis
Diabetes Mellitus	Oral Burning and Itching
Excema and Psoriasis	Oral Lichen Planus
Food Allergies (unexplained)	Rheumatoid Arthritis
Fibromyalgia	Scleroderma
Immune Mediated Pathologies	Sjögren's Syndrome
Lupus Erythematosus	

Mercury Allergy & Relationship to Disease

If you are allergic to mercury and have amalgam fillings, the severity of your allergy will relate directly to the number of amalgam fillings you have and the activities, such as chewing, that stimulate the release of mercury. If you have been suffering from allergic reactions or symptoms that your health professional cannot find a specific cause for, ask him or her to look at mercury as a possible cause or contributor to the problem.

Determining the cause of your allergy takes on even greater importance when it comes to removing your amalgam fillings. Should your doctor conclude that mercury toxicity from dental amalgams may be a contributory factor to your allergies or autoimmune disease, it only makes sense to remove them. However, if you do not have mercury amalgams removed safely, you will be exposing yourself to dangerously high levels of mercury that could trigger a severe allergic reaction.

Because mercury complexes can be allergenic, they can also trigger the onset of autoimmune disease, which is, itself, a type of allergic reaction. When a person develops an autoimmune disease, the immune system mistakenly attacks the body. In the process, it destroys affected cells, organs, and tissues and causes an inflammatory response. When the onset of autoimmune disease is a consequence of mercury toxicity, there is no question that it is a serious consequence, leading some researchers to characterize mercury toxicity as an autoimmune disorder.[11]

Fortunately, the symptoms related to mercury toxicity that are reversible will diminish or disappear completely when the dental amalgam fillings are removed. Improvement is even greater when filling removal is combined with a mercury detoxification program. This evidence will be presented in a later chapter.

CHAPTER 4

Regulatory Standards

"Is elemental mercury escaping from filling material? The answer is an absolute Yes! ... Having worked for OSHA for 17 years, never have I witnessed anything of the magnitude of resistance in acknowledging the danger of toxicity in silver amalgams as by the ADA."
— Dr. Tano Lucero,
Bio-Ethics Medical Center

AGENCIES

The regulatory agencies that monitor occupational safety know that mercury vapor is highly toxic. Because the use of mercury in various industrial processes is a serious health hazard, a number of these agencies have devised guidelines and regulations to protect the health of workers from the effects of mercury poisoning.

The limits that are considered to be harmful, as determined by each agency, differ significantly, in part because of differences in the criteria used to establish permissible levels of exposure. These attempts to establish a safe level for mercury exposure only serve to acknowledge the fact that mercury is a serious health hazard requiring regulatory actions.

Essentially, the principal source of exposure these agencies considered was occupationally related. In setting exposure standards, some of the regulatory agencies assumed that workers are only occupationally exposed to mercury for 40 hours per week. Yet, for millions of people, exposure to mercury from amalgam fillings occurs 24 hours a day, every day of the year. Consequently, current industrial safety standards for mercury do not adequately address all other sources of exposure listed in Table 2-2.

World Health Organization (WHO)

In its evaluation of exposure limits set by various international bodies, WHO has recognized a time-weighted average for occupational exposure to mercury vapor at 25 µg/m³ per eight-hour shift. According to WHO, the damaging effects of exposure to mercury vapor at levels greater than this are well documented; if set higher, the exposure limit would not protect those individuals most sensitive to mercury toxicity—the young, the elderly, pregnant and nursing mothers, and those whose health has already been compromised.[1]

Occupational Safety and Health Administration (OSHA)

The current permissible exposure limit (PEL) to mercury vapor, set by OSHA, is 0.05 mg/m³ or 50 µg/m³ of air, based on an eight-hour work-related exposure for a 40-hour week. While the limit is far more lenient than the WHO standard, OSHA (in a nod toward caution) also set a ceiling limit of 100 µg/m³ of air that is not to be exceeded at any time. If a workplace exceeds this limit of exposure at any time during their shift, employees must leave the area for the remainder of the shift.[2]

National Institute for Occupational Safety and Health (NIOSH)

NIOSH has also established a recommended exposure limit (REL) to mercury vapor at 0.05 mg/m³ or 50 (µg/m³) of air, as a time-weighted average limit of exposure for up to a ten-hour workday and a 40-hour workweek.[3] Like OSHA, NIOSH has added an additional safety ceiling: at no time shall a worker's exposure to mercury vapor exceed 100 µg/m³. The ceiling takes precedence over the time-weighted average; if exposure exceeds this limit, the worker must leave the area. The NIOSH limit is based on the risk of central nervous system damage, as well as eye, skin, and respiratory tract irritation.

NIOSH acknowledges that these safety limits were difficult to establish because a large percentage of the population already presents signs and symptoms of early mercury toxicity similar to what can be observed through such exposure—even though they have not experienced any occupational exposure to mercury. The fact that approximately 80 percent of the U.S. adult population has amalgam fillings suggests that these fillings may be responsible for the high incidence of the low-level toxicity symptoms apparent in the general population. This also suggests that many people who are exposed to mercury in the workplace may *already* exhibit symptoms of mercury poisoning because of their amalgam fillings. For these individuals, the risk of mercury poisoning is significantly elevated.

Agency for Toxic Substances and Disease Registry (ATSDR)

Of all the regulatory bodies, ATSDR takes the most prudent and realistic approach to mercury toxicity. After studying employees who were exposed to 26 $\mu g/m^3$ of mercury vapor for an average of 15.3 years, the agency determined that these employees had a significantly higher percentage of mercury-related symptoms, particularly certain tremors. Allowing for individual variations in sensitivity, ATSDR established a minimal risk level (MRL) for chronic exposure to mercury vapor at 0.2 $\mu g/m^3$ of air. According to the agency, this is the upper limit to which a person can be *continuously* exposed without exhibiting any observable effects.[4] The development of a 24-hour exposure limit makes sense because anyone with amalgam fillings will be exposed to mercury 24 hours a day, seven days a week, regardless of his or her level of mercury exposure in the workplace.

American Conference of Government Industry Hygienists (ACGIH)

ACGIH has assigned mercury vapor a threshold limit value (TLV) of 0.025 mg/m³ or 25 µg/m³ of air as a time-weighted average for a normal 8-hour workday and a 40-hour workweek.[5]

A WIDE VARIANCE

As is evident, the exposure limits for mercury vapor established by the various regulatory agencies show considerable variance: the highest official "safe" level, at 100 µg/m³, is 500 times greater than the lowest, at 0.2 µg/m³. Only the ATSDR guidelines, which are the most conservative of all the agencies' regulations, acknowledge the need for a 24-hour exposure timeframe. In my opinion, it would be prudent for industry to adopt the ATSDR regulations in establishing workplace exposures to mercury vapor.

WHAT IS "SAFE"?

In developing guidelines, regulatory agencies attempt to determine how much mercury the average healthy person can absorb without showing obvious signs of mercury poisoning. However, few agencies consider at-risk individuals, such as nursing mothers or women who are pregnant. Also, they do not consider individuals who have mercury sensitivity or those whose immune systems are compromised. Moreover, they do not consider those hapless souls—and there are millions—who are walking around with a mouthful of mercury.

The agencies themselves acknowledge that it is very difficult to determine a universally safe level because far too many people already show early signs of mercury poisoning. NIOSH, WHO and the U.S. Centers for Disease Control all acknowledge that, practically speaking, there is *no safe level* of mercury exposure.[6-8]

CHAPTER 5

Legislative & Regulatory Initiatives

"The government was concerned over picograms and micrograms of mercury in apples but looked the other way when milligrams, one million times more, were being implanted directly into a child's mouth."
—Dr. Pierre Blais,
Health Canada

The U.S. Occupational Safety and Health Administration (OSHA), the regulatory watchdog for exposure to toxins in the workplace, requires that dental amalgam materials be stored in unbreakable, tightly sealed hazardous waste containers, away from heat. Dental staff must use a "no touch" technique for handling amalgam and no one should handle amalgam material without protection. Moreover, amalgam must be covered with liquid to minimize the release of mercury vapor.[1]

If OSHA has determined that the mercury release from amalgam is of sufficient concern to require special hazardous-substance precautions when handling this material, then why in heaven's name are we putting this stuff in our mouths?

AMALGAM A HAZARDOUS SUBSTANCE—U.S. EPA

The United States Environmental Protection Agency (EPA) now classifies discarded dental amalgam as toxic waste.[2] Under regulations adopted in 1988, any dental office not complying with the requirements for proper handling and disposal of amalgam materials can be fined for contaminating the workplace and the environment. On behalf of the EPA, the U.S Justice Department subsequently sued a group of New England dentists and dental companies for the failure to safely dispose of used amalgam.

> *U.S. EPA: discarded dental amalgams are hazardous waste materials.*

During the proceedings, when the agency was asked whether it considered dental amalgam to be hazardous, the EPA replied that where there is "a release or threatened release of a hazardous substance into the environment ... any substance that contains a listed hazardous substance is *itself* considered to be a hazardous substance."[3] So, if the materials that go into making mercury fillings are considered hazardous *before* they are placed in our teeth, and the fillings are considered to be hazardous waste *after* they have been removed, then why do these same materials mysteriously become nonhazardous when imbedded in our teeth? According to the ADA, amalgams are perfectly safe—obviously, the EPA thinks otherwise.

> *If the materials that go into making mercury fillings are considered hazardous before they are placed in our teeth, and the fillings are considered to be hazardous waste after they have been removed, then why do these same materials mysteriously become nonhazardous when imbedded in our teeth?*

EPA regulations bear many similarities to OSHA regulations: when the components of an amalgam filling—elemental mercury and the powdered metals zinc, silver, tin, and copper—are delivered to the dental office, they must be placed in a hazardous-materials container. Once a dentist removes an amalgam filling from a tooth, the discarded filling particles must be placed in a hazardous-waste container.

MUNICIPAL BYLAWS ENACTED

Nationwide, the U.S. dental profession is the third-largest commercial consumer of mercury and uses tons of mercury every year, most of which ends up in our environment. In fact, amalgam waste from dental offices has been identified as the single largest contributor of mercury into our domestic sewers and sewage treatment plants. When amalgam fillings are removed, approximately 60 percent ends up in the effluent, which is eventually flushed into our lakes and rivers or redistributed on land as treated sludge.

> *Nationwide, the dental profession in the United States is the third-largest commercial consumer of mercury and uses tons of mercury every year, most of which ends up in our environment.*

Consequently, a number of cities throughout the United States and Canada have recently passed bylaws banning the sale, import, or manufacture of mercury products. San Francisco,[4] Seattle's King County,[5] Toronto[6] and Victoria,[7] among others, are now also regulating the discharge of mercury amalgam into sewers.

OTHER REGULATORY INITIATIVES

Banned from house paints by the U.S. EPA since 1990, the elimination of mercury also extends to healthcare. Mercury is now banned or being phased out in virtually all healthcare environments. Mercurochrome, a household disinfectant once widely used for cuts and scrapes, is no longer legal for sale; thermometers and blood pressure kits containing mercury are soon to be a thing of the past; and thimerosal, the ethylmercury preservative used in vaccines, is now on the regulatory chopping block—or so they say.

Ironically, the only discipline that appears to have escaped the sweep of the regulatory broom regarding the use of mercury—and the discipline that continues to be one of the most prolific consumers of this and other toxic metals—is the dental profession.

INDUSTRY DISTANCING ITSELF

The marketplace, however, is certainly getting the message: Dentsply International and Kerr, a subsidiary of Sybron Dental Specialties, two of the largest U.S.-based manufacturers of mercury amalgam materials, now issue warnings regarding potential health hazards. Dentsply's extensive warning label demonstrates a growing recognition that the industry has on its hands a litigative time bomb.

In a long list of precautions that includes contraindications for use in patients with renal deficiency and mercury allergies, children under six, and pregnant women, Dentsply warns that mercury is a skin sensitizer, pulmonary sensitizer, neurotoxin, and nephrotoxin.

The manufacturer cautions that exposure to mercury amalgams may cause:

- irritation to skin, eyes, respiratory tract, and mucous membranes;

- hypersensitivity reactions, allergies, or electrochemically caused local reactions;

- a temporary increase of the mercury concentration in the blood and urine; and

- a galvanic effect, if in contact with other metal restorations.[8]

Also prominent are warnings that:

- the number of amalgam restorations for one patient should be kept to a minimum;

- inhalation of mercury vapor by dental staff should be avoided by proper handling, the use of masks, and proper ventilation;

- contact with skin should be avoided by the use of safety glasses and gloves;

- amalgam scrap must be safely stored in well sealed containers; and

- regulations for disposal must be observed.[9]

One caution, in particular, stands out: "After placement or removal of amalgam restorations, there is a temporary increase of the mercury concentration in the blood and urine."[10] This admission, alone, provides *de facto* recognition by the manufacturers of amalgam materials—contrary to the long-held position of the ADA—that amalgams *do* release mercury into the body and, by implication, add to the cumulative body burden of this known toxin.

There is more: the manufacturer also emphasizes, concentrations [of mercury vapor] as low as 0.03 mg/m^3 "have induced psychiatric symptoms in humans. Renal involvement may be indicated by proteinuria, albuminuria, enzymuria, and anuria. Other effects may include salivation, gingivitis, stomatitis, loosening of the teeth, blue lines on the gums, diarrhea, chronic pneumonitis and mild anemia. Repeated exposure to mercury and its compounds may result in sensitization. Intrauterine exposure may result in tremors and involuntary movements in the infants. Mercury is excreted in breast milk."[11]

Talk about mea culpa—the fact that Dentsply feels compelled to issue such a strong warning about a product it desires to sell speaks volumes about the ADA's disingenuous assurance of safety.

LEGISLATIVE ACTIONS

On the legislative front, passage of the 1997 Colorado dental freedom law, the first of its kind to be enacted in the United States, now assures consumers of their right to choose safe alternatives to conventional dental procedures and provides that mercury-free practitioners can practice without fear of retribution from the ADA and its Colorado affiliate. Enactment of this legislation was a total reversal of a state judiciary decision, made only a year prior, which forbade dentists from removing mercury amalgam and patients from requesting its removal, based on concerns about toxicity.[12]

California Leads the Way

On November 1, 2001, Democratic Representative for the State of California, Diane Watson, set the congressional ball rolling with the introduction of a bill to outlaw the use of amalgam fillings. The bill, which seeks to prohibit the use of amalgam after 2006, is based on the scientific evidence of bioaccumulation of mercury in the fetus and nursing child through maternal placental transmission and breast milk. The bill argues that such restriction is warranted, and is based on the recommendations of the Institute of Medicine and the American Pediatric Association that no product containing mercury should be given to children or pregnant women. Currently, the legislation has been referred to the Committee on House Energy and Commerce, subcommittee on Health.

> *Thimerosal, for generations, has needlessly exposed young children to acute and extremely high levels of mercury.*

Thimerosal Banned

On May 17th, 2004, in a landmark decision that promises to have a domino effect across North America, the State of Iowa set national precedence by banning the use of the potent neurotoxin thimerosal (ethyl mercury) in childhood vaccines.[13] Used as a preservative, thimerosal has been the source of much angry debate between parents, dentists, doctors and scientists. I believe that the current epidemic levels of autism and learning disability may well be a consequence of mercury poisoning from dental amalgams and vaccines.

> *I believe that the current epidemic levels of autism and learning disabilities are the consequence of mercury from dental amalgams and vaccines.*

This is truly a watershed victory for those who have argued that thimerosal, for generations, has needlessly exposed young children to inordinately high levels of mercury. The Iowa initiative should serve as the thin edge of the wedge in the growing public outcry against preventable exposure to mercury from all sources.

International Opposition to Mercury

In several other countries, resistance to the continued use of mercury amalgams has continued to grow. In Great Britain, the ministry of health, after a 1988 review of the evidence of mercury toxicity, directed dentists not to place or remove amalgams during pregnancy.[14] Both Sweden and Canada have also strongly advised against the practice.[15]

In 1991, Sweden declared mercury amalgam to be toxic material "unsuitable for use" and announced the imposition of an outright ban on amalgam fillings. The ban was to be implemented over a ten-year period as suitable replacement materials were found. In a startling public admission, Swedish officials conceded that they erred in allowing mercury amalgam to be used. "We now realize that we have made a mistake. This has caused people to suffer unnecessarily."[16]

> *In 1991, Sweden declared mercury amalgam to be toxic material "unsuitable for use" and announced the imposition of an outright ban on amalgam fillings.*

In 1992, Germany followed suit, prohibiting the sale of conventional gamma-2 amalgams, which are now known to release up to 50 times the level of mercury of previous amalgam formulations. Based on the evidence of prenatal toxicity and demonstrated accumulation of mercury in fetal tissues, Norway joined both Great Britain and Germany in directing dentists to discontinue placing mercury amalgam in pregnant women.

In 1996, *Canadians for Mercury Relief*, a group of Canadian anti-mercury patients, launched legal action to "seek compensation on behalf of Canadians who had mercury amalgams installed without knowing the risk associated with these [amalgam] fillings and also to seek compensation for the many thousands of Canadians who are suffering from the ill effects of mercury poisoning."[17]   The class action suit represents more than 8,000 patients from across Canada. This was followed in 1998 by legal actions against the dental manufacturer Dentsply International and its Canadian division, Johnson & Johnson, and Health Canada. The case is currently awaiting a summary judgment motion.

OTHER INITIATIVES

In 2000, state courts of Maryland ruled that the state's regulatory agency for dentistry violated the law by prohibiting dentists from discussing the risks of mercury amalgam placement with their patients. More recently, Health Canada lowered the recommended exposure limit to mercury from all sources for children and women of child-bearing age. The new limit is 95 percent below the lowest observable adverse effect level (LOAEL) in mercury-sensitive individuals.

ADA OBLIVIOUS TO REALITY

Despite the thousands of clinical cases documenting dramatic improve-ments in the health of individuals who have had their amalgams removed, despite the thousands of peer-reviewed medical references documenting mechanisms by which mercury from amalgam causes degenerative disease,[18] despite the scientific proof that mercury from amalgams accu-mulates in the brain, kidneys, liver and body tissues of everyone who sports a mouth full of metal—and despite the fact that the use of mercury is being banned in jurisdictions throughout the world—the ADA continues to say, "there is no cause for concern."

In a recent article, the *Journal of the American Dental Association*, the official mouthpiece of the ADA, provides the following "insightful" commentary: "Mercury amalgams remain safe and effective. Dentists should educate their patients and other health professionals who may be mistakenly concerned about amalgam safety."[19]

Like the Mad Hatter at Alice's tea party, the ADA's position defies all logic.

CHAPTER 6

Your Mouth—A Toxic Reservoir

"Our laboratory findings in this investigation are at variance with the anecdotal opinion of the dental profession, which claims that amalgam fillings are safe."
—MJ Vimy, et al.,
University of Calgary

According to Dr. Charles Williamson of the Toxic Studies Institute, Boca Raton, Florida, the greatest majority of the body burden of mercury, up to 87 percent, comes from the continuous release of mercury vapor from dental amalgams.[1] Mercury is now listed as Public Enemy #3 on the Top 20 list of toxic substances by the U.S. Agency for Toxic Substance and Disease Registry (ATSDR), surpassed only by arsenic and lead.

OPINIONS IN CONFLICT

The weight of scientific evidence supports the argument that the mercury released from amalgam fillings is a major source of mercury deposited in the body. Research also confirms that once mercury is released, it accumulates in various tissues and organs, damaging or killing cells. However, there is dissenting opinion regarding the relevance of these findings.

A 1988 study, reported in the *Journal of Community Dentistry and Oral Epidemiology* failed to find a significant correlation between the number of fillings and the number of symptoms or prevalence of symptoms. The authors conclude that the results do not support a correlation between the number of fillings and symptoms of toxicity; however, they do not rule out the possibility of such a connection.[2] Similar conclusions have been reached by other researchers.[3-5] More recent studies on serum mercury levels have also failed to find statistically significant correlations between the number of amalgams and health.[6]

This is not surprising. It is well known that blood levels of mercury, while an important measure of transient mercury exposure, are a poor indicator of its cumulative body burden. It is the level of mercury in the *tissues*—not the blood—that prescribes the progression of disease.

STUDIES ON MERCURY EXPOSURE FROM AMALGAMS

Conflicting evidence is not new to scientific inquiry. While Mother Nature has never been known to reveal herself easily, her coquettish ways certainly do complicate the process. That said, the evidence existing today *is* irrefutable:

- Mercury, in all its forms, is a powerful poison.

- Mercury is continually released from amalgam fillings.

- The release of mercury from amalgam results in a cumulative rise of the poison in body tissues, particularly in the kidneys and the CNS.

- There is no established safe level of mercury.

Numerous studies demonstrate that inorganic mercury, including particulate matter, is released from dental amalgams *in vitro* (in the laboratory).[7,8] Other studies confirm that mercury vapor released *in vivo* (in the body) leads to an increased uptake of the metal in body tissues.[9-13] Canadian researchers, investigating the release of mercury vapor following amalgam stimulation, found that the level of mercury spikes dramatically when amalgam is stimulated and remains elevated during the course of chewing, declining slowly over 90 minutes following cessation of chewing.[14] The dosages recorded were as much as 18 times the allowable daily limits established by some countries for mercury exposure from all sources. According to the authors, the results demonstrate that the amount of elemental mercury vapor released from dental amalgam exceeds a major percentage of internationally accepted threshold limits for environmental mercury exposure.

Granted, making accurate quantitative assessments of the amount of mercury released from amalgams and subsequently absorbed by the body can be difficult.[15-7] Nevertheless, the published data demonstrate that the probability is high of developing classical neurological symptoms of chronic mercury poisoning, including tremors, proteinuria (excessive protein in the urine) and erethism (excessive irritability and sensitivity to stimuli), when exposure to mercury vapor exceeds 80 $\mu g/m^3$ of air. Exposure in the range of 25 to 80 $\mu g/m^3$ is less severe and the effects are generally present only in sensitive individuals. These include defects in psychomotor performance, tremors, fatigue, irritability, and loss of appetite.

As demonstrated by the work of Vimy and Lorscheider,[18] the release of mercury vapor from the stimulation of amalgams by chewing can temporarily exceed 30 $\mu g/m^3$ of air—well above the level where harmful effects in sensitive individuals have been demonstrated. At intake levels of 10 to 30 μg of mercury per day, other researchers report adverse changes in thyroid uptake, liver and cardiovascular function, adrenal gland activity and immunologic responses. Several studies also note an association between the number of amalgam fillings and the resident mercury content in the brain and kidneys.

Using kidney and brain tissue from autopsies, Swedish researchers found a high correlation between the number of tooth surfaces containing amalgam and the concentration of mercury in the occipital cortex of the brain.[19] The same study showed that the amount of mercury in the kidneys of amalgam carriers was almost ten-fold higher than the

A comparative study of dental staff exposed to mercury vapor revealed exceedingly high levels of mercury in the pituitary glands, more than thirty-five times that of the nonoccupational control group.

amount of mercury in amalgam-free individuals. As well, a comparative study of dental staff exposed to mercury vapor revealed exceedingly high levels of mercury in the pituitary glands, more than thirty-five times that of the nonoccupational control group.[20]

Other researchers report mercury concentrations in the grey and white matter of brain tissue of amalgam users that were approximately two to three times that of amalgam-free individuals.[21,22] While recognizing the fact that the toxic levels of mercury in the brain have not been sufficiently investigated to determine clinical significance, the authors conclude that their research provides strong evidence that mercury from amalgam fillings contributes to the body burden of mercury in the brain.

Studies conducted on animals confirm the deposition of mercury in body tissues. Researchers at the University of Calgary placed radioactive mercury-203 amalgam fillings in the teeth of adult sheep.[23] Using a whole-body radiometric scanning technique, within days the radioactive isotope appeared in several tissues and organs, exhibiting particularly high concentrations in the kidneys and liver.

In a more detailed study, Vimy and coworkers used similar methods to follow the uptake of mercury released from amalgams placed in the teeth of pregnant ewes. Mercury appeared in the maternal and fetal blood and the amniotic fluid within two days after placement of amalgam tooth restorations. All examined tissues displayed mercury accumulation, with the highest adult concentrations in the kidney and liver. Fetal concentrations in the liver and pituitary gland were exceptionally high[24] —a worrisome finding made more so with the revelation that the placenta appeared to progressively concentrate mercury with the advance of gestation. The authors state, "Our laboratory findings in this investigation are at variance with the anecdotal opinion of the dental profession, which claims that amalgam fillings are safe."[25]

> *Mercury originating from maternal amalgam fillings transfers across the placenta to the fetus. It also enters the breast milk ingested by the newborn and ultimately into the infant's body tissues.*

In an investigation of lactating women with aged amalgam fillings, increased mercury excretion in the breast milk and urine correlated with the number of fillings and mercury vapor concentrations in the oral cavity.[26] The authors concluded that mercury originating from maternal amalgam fillings transfers across the placenta to the fetus. It also enters the breast milk ingested by the newborn, and ultimately into the infant's body tissues. The implications of these findings have great relevance for women of child-bearing years.

Benefits of Amalgam Removal

Studies conducted on removal of amalgams have shown encouraging results with respect to body mercury levels. In one investigation on blood and tissue mercury levels following amalgam removal, researchers found a statistically significant drop in blood levels at 18 weeks. Although removal of the amalgams provided an additional transient exposure, the added mercury burden was rapidly cleared from the blood with a half-life of 2.9 days.[27]

In another study, evaluation of tissue mercury levels following replacement of mercury amalgams with gold inlays revealed that, despite a significant but transient elevation of blood and urinary mercury immediately following amalgam removal, plasma and urinary mercury levels were markedly reduced within twelve months of removal to 50 percent and 25 percent, respectively, of the initial values.[28]

Similar findings have been confirmed in other recent studies.[29,30] Berglund and coworkers report a significant drop in body mercury burden following amalgam removal. The researchers also found that the use of a rubber dam during removal of amalgam restorations significantly reduced the transient elevation of mercury that followed removal.[31]

MERCURY VAPOR ANALYZER

The mercury vapor analyzer, the instrument of choice to evaluate mercury vapor in the workplace, allows an apples-to-apples comparison of the amount of mercury considered safe and the amount that amalgam fillings release. Using the mercury vapor analyzer, researchers have shown that, under certain types of stimulation, amalgams can release up to 200 times more mercury vapor than unstimulated fillings—and far more than is permissible under current regulatory standards.

As long as amalgam fillings are in your mouth, they are slowly but relentlessly releasing mercury vapor. Consequently, a significant portion of the population, perhaps including you, could easily exceed the daily "safe" eight-hour levels of exposure solely from what is released from their amalgam fillings.

Based on WHO standards, if more than 25 µg of mercury are released from amalgam fillings every hour for 8 hours, that person's mouth is "unsafe." By ATSDR standards, if the amount of mercury released from a person's amalgam fillings exceeds an average of 0.2 µg/m^3 over a 24-hour period, that person's mouth becomes an "unsafe" environment. The amount of mercury that amalgam fillings release into the oral cavity can range from 3 µg/m^3 to over 4295 µg/m^3. Unfortunately, when mercury from this source exceeds "safe" levels, people with amalgam fillings cannot leave the contaminated area. The only way to insure your mouth is a safe environment is to have your fillings removed. Then you need to deal with the mercury stored in your body.

Determining Factors

A number of factors must be considered in order to determine how much mercury vapor amalgam fillings release every day. The amount discharged is related to the degree of amalgam stimulation. Stimulation is any activity that exacerbates the release of mercury vapor or the fracturing of particles from fillings, including: heat, abrasion, compression, chemical and electro-chemical stimulation; and the possible release from exposure to electro-magnetic fields, such as cellular telephones and microwaves.

Two people of the same age and the same state of health, who have an identical number of amalgams, will not necessarily release the same amount of mercury over a 24-hour period. The differences relate to daily habits and activities, which are highly variable. People who chew gum constantly, snack throughout the day, frequently drink hot liquids, grind their teeth and breathe through their mouth, will be exposed to much more mercury than those who do not engage in these activities. These individual differences can be substantial and may account for much of the difficulty in correlating mercury exposure to the number and size of amalgams.

What the Mercury Vapor Analyzer Reveals

At *Sanoviv Medical Institute*, the dental department uses the *Jerome*®
mercury vapor analyzer, manufactured by Arizona Instruments, to measure the mercury vapor that is released when a patient with amalgam fillings brushes his or her teeth. The procedure is as follows:

The patient avoids any stimulation of the fillings for two hours before
testing. A prestimulation oral air sample is then taken. This sample normally shows a low reading because fillings generally release much smaller
amounts of mercury when they are not stimulated.

The patient then brushes the surfaces of the amalgam fillings for ten seconds,
using a soft-bristle toothbrush with no toothpaste, and the *Jerome*® analyzer
is used to test for mercury vapor immediately following stimulation.

Using this procedure, we have recorded oral mercury vapor levels as high
as 400 µg/m³. Readings in excess of 999 µg/m³ of mercury have been
recorded when extracted teeth with amalgam fillings were brushed for the
same period of time.

To show what amounts of mercury are released over time, we take readings at ten-minute intervals for a 90-minute period. Each reading shows
the continued presence of mercury, with the amounts decreasing over
time. The amount of mercury that brushing releases varies, depending
on the number of fillings, the type of amalgam used, the size of the filling,
the amount of saliva present, and whether gold fillings are also present.
The presence of excess saliva often results in a lower reading because
saliva can capture some of the mercury vapor. While this sounds advan-
tageous, keep in mind that any mercury vapor that is captured by saliva,
liquids, or foods will be converted to methylmercury in the mouth and
the intestine. This organic form of mercury is more toxic than elemental mercury and is readily absorbed into the body.

Several other researchers have examined how much mercury is released
from fillings during various forms of stimulation. In a study by
Malmström and coworkers,[32] subjects had their amalgam fillings stimulated by the various modes listed below. The following table shows
the results.

Table 6-1

Stimulation of Amalgam Fillings

Stimulant	Mercury Released ($\mu g/m^3$)
Amalgam Fillings at Rest	36
Chewing Food	68
Eating Sweets	70
Tooth Brushing	272
Polishing Filling after a Dental Cleaning*	504
Wet Polishing an Amalgam Filling*	597
Dry Polishing an Amalgam Filling*	4295

Stimulation initiated at a dental office.
From Malmstrom, C., Danish Dental Journal, October 1989.

Even though a mercury vapor analyzer cannot tell you where the mercury will end up in your body or what specific damage it will cause, it provides *prima facia* evidence that mercury is released from amalgam fillings. The analyzer also proves that different types of stimulation release different amounts of mercury vapor. It is important to understand that the release of mercury is increased every time fillings are stimulated, and continues to be released at this higher level until the stimulation has ceased and the filling has cooled.

> *The release of mercury is increased every time fillings are stimulated, and continues to be released at this higher level until the stimulation has ceased and the filling has cooled.*

Another factor affecting the release of mercury from amalgams is the presence of other metals in the oral cavity. If both mercury amalgams and gold crowns are present, or gold crowns have been laid over an amalgam (a common occurrence), the differences in the electrolytic potential of the two metals creates a galvanic current. In the moist environment of the oral cavity, this current is constant and will cause the filling to release a significantly higher level of mercury—even when the amalgam is not stimulated.

In conclusion, the evidence presented through thousands of animal and clinical studies, and verified with the mercury vapor analyzer, is unassailable: amalgam fillings discharge mercury. Sometimes they release a little, sometimes they release a lot; it all depends on how frequently and how aggressively they are stimulated. The findings totally belie the dental industry's claim that, once mercury is mixed with other metals, it is safely locked inside the amalgam.

The more pertinent question remains: "If my amalgams are leaking mercury and if that mercury vapor is being absorbed by my body, is there anything I can do about it?"

CHAPTER 7

Into the Mouths of Babes

"Seven million women throughout the United States have so much mercury in their systems that pregnancy would pose a serious threat to the developing fetus."
— Tom McGuire, DDS.,
citing a study from the CDC

In 1986, the State of California passed the *Safe Drinking Water and Toxic Enforcement Act* (Proposition 65). The act, designed to protect pregnant women and their unborn children from chemicals with demonstrated carcinogenic or reproductive toxicity, lists many chemicals, several dozen of which—including mercury—are used in dental materials and treatments. The act further specifies that no person or company may

"Once mothers realize the fillings in their teeth damage the development of their babies' brains while they're in the womb, and once these women understand this damage can result in low IQ, learning and behavioral problems after birth, then we'll see a public outcry against the use of mercury amalgam."
— Dr. Charles Williamson,
Toxic Studies Institute

expose a person to any substance listed in the act without prior warning. While it has been in place for years, Proposition 65, until recently, has been willfully ignored by the dental industry and practicing dentists.

In 1991, a group of dentists filed suit against the ADA, claiming fraud and negligence against the association in its misrepresentation of the facts regarding amalgam's adverse effects. The plaintiff's claim was that the actions of the ADA had harmed the doctor-patient relationship and endangered public health.[1] In 1993, a California-based consumer advocacy group, the Environmental Law Foundation, and a Washington-based organization, Consumers for Dental Choice, served violation notices under provisions of Proposition 65 against several dental amalgam manufacturers for their failure to inform the public about mercury toxicity. At that time, such public warnings were in common use in several countries, including all those of the European Union.[2]

The initiative was fought so vigorously by the ADA and its California affiliate that the Governor of the State of California, finding their stalling tactics entirely reprehensible, summarily dismissed all ADA representatives from the State Dental Board and replaced them with a new delegation.[3] In 1999, the revised board labeled mercury a hazardous material and directed dentists to warn their patients about its toxicity to mother and fetus. This was followed in 2001 by a second legal challenge when, As You Sow, another U.S.-based environmental group, sued 80 California dentists under the provisions of Proposition 65 for continued disregard of the need to inform the public of the dangers of mercury.

Despite the efforts of amalgam manufacturers and the ADA to derail the issue of mercury toxicity, a formal judgment was passed in 2003 requiring all dental offices in California to post the following warning: *"Dental amalgams, used in many dental offices, causes exposure to mercury, a chemical known to the State of California to cause birth defects or other reproductive harm."*[4] While a small step, the victory has proven to be a significant milestone for consumers' rights: California is the first U.S. state to require dentists to inform their patients about the toxic nature of mercury in amalgam fillings.

PROTECTING MOTHER AND CHILD

On the global stage, the World Health Organization (WHO), already on record in recognizing amalgam fillings as the greatest source of mercury exposure in humans, further acknowledges the particular vulnerability of the fetus and newborn to mercury toxicity. The WHO review of the environmental health effects of inorganic mercury, published in 1991, documents several animal studies that indicate increased frequencies of spontaneous abortions, low birth weights, malformations, cardiac abnormalities and other congenital defects following maternal exposure to mercury.[5] Similar studies on human maternal exposure indicate similar fetal response patterns.

> *The cumulative effect of mercury amalgam poisoning makes it one of the most serious health hazards facing Americans today—particularly our children and young souls yet to be born.*

According to the U.S. Centers for Disease Control (CDC), heavy metals, such as mercury, arsenic and lead, top the list of global environmental threats to children. The CDC has recently estimated that seven million women throughout the United States have so much mercury in their systems that pregnancy would pose a serious threat to the developing fetus.[6] According to the Toxic Element Research Foundation (TERF), the cumulative effect of mercury amalgam poisoning makes it one of the most serious health hazards facing Americans today—particularly our children and young souls yet to be born.

PLEASE BE CAREFUL, GOD ISN'T FINISHED WITH ME YET

The scientific studies regarding children are even more conclusive where mercury poisoning is concerned. Researchers caution that adult analyses are simply inapplicable to children, who are demonstrably more sensitive to amalgam.[7] Moreover, because mercury exposure can give rise to allergic reactions and immunological responses which may be genetically regulated, it has not been possible to establish a level of mercury in the blood or urine *below* which mercury-related toxicity symptoms will not occur.[8] In short, any exposure to mercury—no matter how small—may prove harmful to sensitive individuals.

Several studies confirm that mercury can pass from the blood of the mother through the placenta and into the fetus. A recent clinical assessment of a pregnant woman accidentally exposed to mercury vapor revealed comparable levels of the toxin in the blood of mother and infant at birth and six days later. The findings disclose a free transfer of mercury across the placenta.[9] Likewise, a German study, designed to measure mercury contamination from amalgams and other sources, found a striking correlation between the levels of mercury in mothers and their newborn infants.[10]

Because the fetus and newborn are dramatically more susceptible to toxic substances than adults, significantly smaller amounts of any toxin can disrupt growth and development, particularly before birth. During the first trimester of pregnancy, the fetus undergoes astounding growth as the genetically programmed process of cell differentiation choreographs the intricate development of specialized tissues and organs. Because the important antioxidant and detoxification systems responsible for removing toxic materials are not yet developed, the fetus remains extremely vulnerable during this critical phase of growth.[11]

Animal studies show that a primary fetal site for accumulation of mercury from maternal amalgams is the liver. Following birth, the infant continues to receive amalgam mercury from the mother's milk.[12] The level of mercury in the fetus is directly proportional to the number of amalgam surfaces in the mother's mouth: the more fillings a mother has, the greater will be the exposure to the fetus.[13] The toxin crosses the placental barrier with ease, concentrating in fetal tissues at levels almost twice that of the mother. Unlike the comparable blood levels of mercury between fetus and mother noted earlier, fetal tissue demonstrates a distinct propensity to concentrate the poison—much to the detriment of the fetus.

Exposure of the fetus to mercury decreases the flow of oxygen and vital nutrients, including amino acids, glucose, magnesium, zinc, and vitamin B_{12}, and depresses the activity of critical enzyme systems. This can lead to retardation in development, particularly with respect to the central nervous system.[14]

Mercury Exposure During Pregnancy

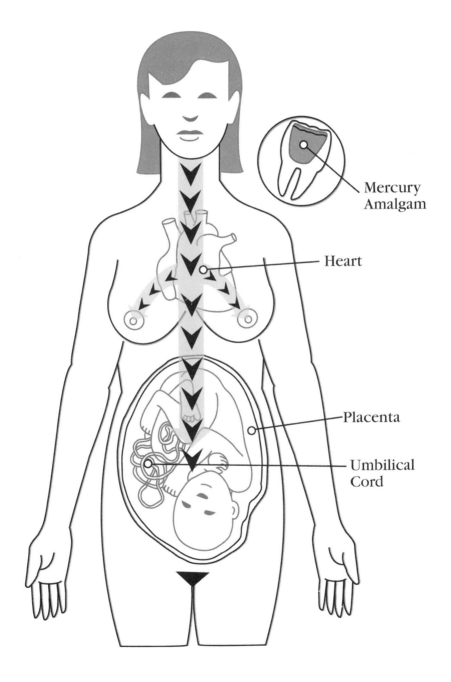

Mercury
Amalgam

Heart

Placenta

Umbilical
Cord

Unfortunately, fetal mercury poisoning problems can be compounded ten-fold when a pregnant woman has amalgams placed or removed during the first trimester of pregnancy.[15] Acute exposure of the fetus to high levels of maternal mercury from amalgam placement or removal can be devastating because the critical liver detoxifications systems are not fully developed until well after birth.

GENETIC, NEUROLOGICAL AND HORMONAL ABERRATIONS

Mercury can alter the genetic blueprint or DNA within the cells of the developing embryo and fetus. Results of animal studies have shown that even extremely low doses of methylmercury can severely inhibit cell division and induce chromosomal breakage. Of greatest concern is mercury's well documented ability to cause genetic mutations[16,17] leading to birth defects[18] and learning disabilities.[19,20]

Exposure of the fetus to mercury can also cause serious disruption in brain development, involving a reduction in total brain mass, loss of neurons, and developmental imbalances.[21] The consequences include attention deficit disorder ADD,[22] behavioral disorders, a lowering of the intelligence quotient (IQ), and mental retardation.[23]

Because the blood-brain barrier (which provides some protection against mercury toxicity in the adult) is not yet developed at the fetal stage, mercury and other toxic substances to which the mother may be exposed have direct access to the developing brain. It is here, at the "hard-wiring" stage, that powerful poisons, such as mercury, can have their most profound effect. When it comes to fetal neurological development, exposure of mother and fetus to mercury can cut short young dreams before they are even formed.

> *It is at the "hard-wiring" stage that powerful toxins, such as mercury, can have their most profound effect. Toxic exposure of mother and fetus to mercury can cut short young dreams before they are even formed.*

Autism, a complex developmental disability that typically appears during the first three years of life, may have a direct connection with early exposure to mercury.[24] Some researchers suggest that amalgam fillings could be a large part of the reason for the explosion of learning problems, including autism and attention deficit disorder (ADD), since World War II—a time corresponding to the first widespread use of mercury amalgam.[25] In Great Britain, concern regarding the effect of mercury poisoning on the development of intelligence has recently led to the launch of a five-year children's amalgam trial: the study will compare mercury amalgam placement to the use of mercury-free materials and their relative effects on IQ and cognitive development.[26]

It is known that mercury concentrates in the fetal pituitary gland, the body's master gland, which plays a major role in the development of the immune system.[27] Fetal and early childhood exposure to mercury may contribute to a weakened or poorly functioning immune system, making the infant much more susceptible to disease in adulthood. Moreover, toxic damage to the pituitary in early development may lead to the malfunctioning of the entire endocrine and reproductive systems later in life, causing profound hormonal and reproductive disturbances.

Methylmercury and the Nursing Mother

Both before and after birth, the child can be exposed to the most dangerous form of mercury—methylmercury. This organic form of mercury is produced from bacteria resident in the oral cavity and the intestine, which can convert the elemental mercury vapor, released from amalgams, into this decidedly more toxic organic form. Estimated to be one-hundred times more poisonous than elemental mercury, methylmercury is about 1,000-fold more effective in causing genetic damage than is colchicine, the next most potent mutagenic agent known. Most alarming, pregnant women who show no signs of mercury poisoning can give birth to a child with severe neurological disorders that can be traced to mercury or methylmercury toxicity.[28] We know that methylmercury can harm every part of the body and, like elemental mercury, can cross the blood-brain barrier, where it accumulates at levels 30 percent higher in the fetus than in the mother, to inflict serious and permanent brain and neurological damage.[29]

A recent study of methylmercury and inorganic mercury in the blood and urine of pregnant and lactating women exposed to the metal showed that the level of methylmercury in the blood of the umbilical cord (which nourishes the fetus) was almost twice the level of the mother's blood. As well, inorganic and total mercury in the blood were highly correlated with the number of maternal amalgam fillings. The same study demonstrated that maternal mercury concentrations decreased during lactation, likely due to excretion of the toxin into the milk, which is then consumed by the nursing infant.[30] As the milk is digested, mercury enters the child's blood stream and crosses the still undeveloped blood-brain barrier, concentrating in the developing brain and central nervous system.

> *Removal of mercury amalgams well before conception will eliminate a potent source of toxicity for your child. DO NOT consider removal if you are already pregnant or nursing.*

Moreover, tissue levels of mercury in nursing infants and developing children have also been found to be directly related to the number of maternal amalgam fillings.[31-34] The level of exposure to the fetus is dependent on numerous factors, including: 1) the type and amount of mercury; 2) the duration of exposure; 3) age at first exposure; 4) the health and diet of the mother, and 5) her daily habits that stimulate release of mercury from amalgams. Because tissue levels of mercury in the fetus can double those of the mother, the total body burden at birth can be considerable— a tragic way for a child to enter this world.

If you are a female of child-bearing years and have a mouth full of mercury, seriously consider your options. Unquestionably, removal of mercury amalgams well before conception will eliminate a potent source of toxicity for your child. However, do not—DO NOT—consider removal of amalgams if you are already pregnant or nursing. Unless appropriate protective measures are taken, transient but dramatic elevations of mercury are unavoidable. Removal of amalgams in an unsafe way is a toxic event of the highest magnitude and must be avoided prior to and during pregnancy. The key here is to have them removed as many months as possible before conception.

I'm Too Little to Take This

The mercury threat can be compounded with a child's first visit to the dentist. German researchers, in 1994, discovered that children with amalgam fillings had a four-fold higher urinary mercury level than did children without amalgams.[35] Moreover, the level of mercury correlated with the number and extent of the children's fillings. This finding has been confirmed in several other studies. In one recent investigation, children with no previous amalgams showed marked increases in urinary mercury levels following amalgam placement.[36] Interestingly, a recent German study has recorded a marked decrease in the overall body burden of mercury in children over the last ten years, a consequence attributed to the mandated decline in the use of mercury amalgams in that country.[37]

While not as vulnerable as the fetus or nursing infant, children remain far more susceptible than adults to toxins such as mercury.[38] Once they receive their own amalgam fillings, children may exhibit signs of mercury toxicity, especially if they received significant exposure from their mother while in the womb and while nursing.

The pituitary gland is a critical pathway for the transport of mercury from the oral cavity to the brain of a child who has amalgam fillings. The vapor has an extremely high affinity for the gland, penetrating the soft, bony plate in the roof of the nasal cavity and migrating along the neurons to reach the brain. The effects of mercury exposure on children can be extensive and can involve the entire cortex and frontal area, with a consequent reduction in brain mass and functional neurons.[39]

THIMEROSAL IN VACCINES

Another threat of mercury toxicity comes from a source we normally regard as a preventive measure against health problems—vaccinations for infectious diseases. Concern about exposure to mercury and the possible links to autism and other health effects in children prompted the Institute of Medicine (IOM), in 2001, to recommend that all vaccinations containing the preservative thimerosal be removed from shelves and immediately destroyed.[40]

Thimerosal undoubtedly leads to an increase in a child's overall body burden of mercury. Each vaccination preserved with thimerosal will

inject as much as 237 micrograms of mercury into a child's body—
equivalent to milligram doses of mercury for an adult. When you consider
that a child could easily have 16 or more vaccinations by his or her fifth
year, it is easy to see that the level of mercury exposure through vaccination can be staggering.

The recent landmark decision by the State of Iowa to ban the use of
thimerosal in vaccines, as discussed earlier, is a positive development that
promises to have far-reaching effects in eliminating the senseless use of
this poison.

Consumption of Fish during Pregnancy

Gynecologists are now counseling couples who are planning to have a
family not to consume fish during the woman's pregnancy. This caution
concurs with the U.S. Food and Drug Administration's (FDA) advice to
limit consumption of certain seafoods to no more than once a month.
Shark, Mediterranean tuna, swordfish, mackerel and tilefish have all been
shown to have much higher levels of methylmercury than other commonly
eaten fish. This warning takes on more importance when you realize
that the fetus is more susceptible than the mother to the adverse effects
of methylmercury. The FDA extends this advice to pregnant and nursing
women and women who are planning to have children, especially since
dietary practices immediately before pregnancy have a direct bearing on
fetal exposure during the first trimester.

There is a great irony here: while the government advises women of
child-bearing age to limit their consumption of fish that contain mercury,
amalgam fillings can expose these same women to significantly greater
amounts of mercury. Such exposure is not once a month; it occurs all
day, every day. Yet, with exception of a few progressive states that have
recognized the dangers of mercury toxicity, there are no restrictions on
who can have amalgam fillings, how many they can have, or when the
fillings can be placed. Of all the sources of mercury exposure a growing
child will face, by far the greatest body burden—87 percent—will
come from the elemental mercury released from the mother's amalgams
during gestation.

The insidious thing about mercury poisoning is that it is a "retention
toxicity," meaning that its effects are progressive and cumulative.

Depending on the rate of assimilation in the tissues, its effects may not show up for years, perhaps decades. In addition, the symptoms mimic so many other disease processes that a definitive diagnosis is exceedingly difficult to obtain. That is why mercury poisoning has become known as the "Great Masquerader."

There is one thing, however, of which you can be certain. If you were born to a mother with amalgam fillings and you now have fillings yourself, you have been slowly but persistently accumulating mercury in your body since conception. In addition, if your mother was conscientious and made sure that you received all of your requisite vaccinations, it is likely that your present body burden of mercury is considerable.

> *If you were born to a mother with amalgam fillings and you now have fillings yourself, you have been slowly but persistently accumulating mercury in your body since conception.*

Do the Right Thing

If you are a mother, or plan to become one soon, you carry a great responsibility in your deliberation about what to do with your amalgam fillings. I urge you to remember, you will not only be making the decision for yourself, but also for your baby. Like every mother, you will want to do what is best to provide your child with every opportunity to succeed in life. Please, do not jeopardize that future by exposing your child to mercury during the most critical stages of development. Rest assured, a child who has never been exposed to mercury from maternal amalgam fillings will be far healthier than one whose development was compromised by this treacherous poison.

The decision is yours—do the right thing.

CHAPTER 8

Mechanisms of Mercury Toxicity

The information in this chapter may be too technical for some readers. I felt compelled, however, to present it, since this information is not readily available. It is not essential for an understanding of the health threat of amalgams. If it is not of interest to you please fast forward to Chapter 9.

Mercury, in any form or amount, will damage or kill any cell in the body with which it comes into contact. It is a systemic assassin, so poisonous that its presence in the body leaves a virtual killing field of destruction.

For a toxin to be so potent and pervasive, it must act at a fundamental level common to all cells. In the case of mercury, the metal's solubility in fats gives it a special affinity for those tissues and organs that have a high lipid (fat) content. These include: the kidneys; the brain and spinal cord; the liver; and the glandular tissues of the pancreas, testes, ovaries and prostate.

Understanding the mechanisms of toxicity within these target organs can provide a better understanding of the confusing kaleidoscope of symptoms associated with mercury toxicity. It also helps to clarify why patients with seemingly disparate neurological, immunological and systemic disorders (including rheumatoid arthritis, fibromyalgia, eczema, chronic fatigue syndrome, multiple sclerosis, lupus, amyotrophic lateral sclerosis, thyroiditis, glomerulonephritis, and emotional/mood disorders), often improve significantly or recover completely after mercury is removed from the body.

The nature of mercury toxicity can be categorized into three principal effects on the body:

1. systemic;
2. immunological; and
3. neurological.

SYSTEMIC

The pervasive nature of mercury toxicity is characterized by the multitude of effects that the poison has on virtually every aspect of the body. Mercury can disrupt both structure and function from the cellular level to the level of organs and systems.

Cellular Disruptions

Mercury binds with proteins on the surfaces of cell membranes, disrupting the transport of materials in and out of cells and causing them to become "leaky." This is particularly damaging to the cells of the blood-brain barrier, where such damage facilitates the penetration of other toxic substances into the CNS,[1] thereby enhancing the overall toxic challenge.

Mercury interferes with cellular respiration by disrupting the production of ATP that takes place within the mitochondria, tiny organelles that are the powerhouses of the cell. Through these actions, mercury deprives the cell of its ability to replenish vital ATP stores. This systemic interference with cellular energy production explains the profound fatigue often experienced with mercury poisoning. I believe that interference with ATP production by the poisoning of critical respiratory enzymes with mercury is a major contributor to chronic fatigue syndrome.

> *I believe that interference with ATP production by the poisoning of critical respiratory enzymes with mercury is a major contributor to chronic fatigue syndrome.*

Blood and Circulation

By binding aggressively to the oxygen-carrying sites of hemoglobin, molecules that transport oxygen in red blood cells, mercury reduces the ability of the circulatory system to deliver oxygen to the tissues and further diminishes the energy available to the body. In addition, the metal has been found to destroy red blood cell membranes and damage the lining of blood vessels. Its accumulation in the heart also damages the heart muscle and the valves, which regulate blood flow.

These effects account for the noted irregularities in blood hemoglobin and evidence of chest pains and tachycardia (abnormally rapid heart beat) in cases of mercury poisoning. Mercury levels in the heart tissues of individuals who have died from idiopathic dilated cardiomyopathy (IDCM)—many of whom were well-conditioned athletes who dropped dead during sporting events—have been found to contain mercury levels 22,000 times that of individuals who died of other forms of heart disease.[2]

Protein Damage

The ability of mercury to bind to sulfhydryl (SH) groups, common to some amino acids, results in the inhibition of sulfur-containing enzymes and deformation of proteins. Enzyme inactivation is now believed to be the principal means by which mercury poisoning contributes to the development of allergic responses such as in autism, schizophrenia and scleroderma. Formation of strong bonds with -SH groups also causes excessive release of calcium from the mitochondria and reduces the availability of glutathione, a critically important antioxidant and detoxicant in the body. The consequences to the cell are devastating. These processes knock critical metabolic pathways out of commission, disrupt cellular structures, and poison the cell with toxic mercury-sulfur complexes.

Oxidative Stress

Mercury poisoning impairs the ability of cells to manufacture superoxide dismutase (SOD), an antioxidant enzyme vital to the general health of the cell and responsible for neutralizing superoxide free radicals. A study investigating the production of free radicals following exposure to mercury, conducted by researchers at the National Center for Toxicological

> *The disturbing ability of mercury to destroy critical antioxidant enzymes is further magnified by its ability to deplete the body of several minerals essential for proper enzyme function.*

Research, noted a significant loss of SOD activity in the cerebellum, the region of the brain responsible for muscular coordination. The investigators also found that the activity of glutathione peroxidase, an antioxidant enzyme that controls another critical detoxification pathway, was inhibited in both the cerebellum and the brain stem. The findings led the authors to conclude that oxidative stress related to mercury poisoning is a major contributor to the development of neurodegenerative disorders.[4] Similar findings also reveal impairment of other antioxidant enzymes in the blood as a consequence of oxidative damage caused by chronic mercury exposure.[5]

The disturbing ability of mercury to destroy critical antioxidant enzymes is magnified by its ability to deplete the body of several minerals essential for proper enzyme function. Through these actions, mercury effectively antagonizes and diminishes the body's antioxidant and detoxification mechanisms.[6,7]

As a pro-oxidant, mercury's ability to generate free radicals is prodigious and also results in an increase in the production of advanced glycation end products (AGEs). Apart from their ability to degrade cellular function and accelerate the aging process, these troublesome protein/sugar complexes cause certain nerve cells in the brain to pump out superoxide free radicals. Free-radical oxidation, in turn, increases the formation of AGEs, creating a vicious cycle which leads to cell death. The substantia nigra, a region of the brain which manufactures the neurotransmitter dopamine,

is susceptible to AGE-related oxidative damage. Loss of dopamine production in the hippocampus results in a profound degradation of voluntary
control and has been shown to be the likely cause of Parkinson's disease.

IMMUNOLOGICAL

Mercury exposure, even at very low levels, diminishes the ability of the
immune system to meet the slightest challenge. This appears to be a consequence of the metal's ability to depress the number of T lymphocytes
(T cells) in the blood. T cells, one of the body's front-line defenses
against infection, are white blood cells which attack entities that the body
recognizes as invaders.

The number of T cells in the blood declines markedly when amalgam is
placed in the teeth, and they have been found to undergo a programmed
cellular death (*apoptosis*) in the presence of mercury.[8] Alteration of the
ratio of two types of T cells in the blood as a consequence of insertion of
amalgam fillings[9] is now believed to play a central role in the development of several diseases related to suppression of the immune system.
These include lupus, inflammatory bowel syndrome, anemia, multiple
sclerosis and eczema.

Mercury also appears to impair the function of neutrophils, another type
of white blood cell important in the response to infection. Workers
exposed to moderate levels of mercury were found to have impaired
resistance to infections such as *Candida albicans*, a recurring yeast
infection that can spread throughout the body.[10] *Candida*, in turn,
causes a conversion of mercury into an extremely toxic organic form,
which can cross the blood-brain barrier and accumulate in the brain.
Through depression of the immune system and its promotion of
Candida infections, mercury exposure from amalgam may be another
contributing factor to the development of chronic fatigue syndrome.

Mercury has been shown to impair other immune cells, such as the B
lymphocytes and macrophages, which work together to seek out and
destroy invading organisms. The metal also interferes with the production
of antibodies and of cytokines, specialized proteins that prompt the white
blood cells to swing into action, thus crippling the immune system's early
warning defense and exposing the body to enhanced viral infections.[11,12]

By reducing the ability of cells to manufacture antibodies and the antiviral protein, Interferon, mercury degrades the capacity of the immune system to block the spread of bacterial and viral infections to other cells. This leaves the individual susceptible to opportunistic infections.[13] From common challenges, such as *Herpes simplex*, a virus which causes fever blisters and cold sores, to *Chlamidia trachomatis* and other sexually transmitted diseases (STDs), the individual burdened with a heavy accumulation of mercury remains much more vulnerable.

In addition to depressing immune resistance at low levels of exposure, mercury also triggers the release of the inflammatory cytokines Interleukin I (IL-1) and Tumor Necrosis Factor (TNF) in joint tissue.[14] Both proteins are manufactured by white blood cells and play an active role in acute inflammation. Chronic stimulation of IL-1 and TNF can cause cartilage damage and bone destruction and also contributes to cardiovascular disease.

Autoimmune Responses

Glomerulonephritis (inflammation of the kidney) results in an acute autoimmune response in which the body attacks itself; it is perhaps the most insidious effect of early mercury toxicity. It is believed that mercury attaches to the surfaces of cells of the glomeruli, the microscopic filtering structures in the kidney. Thinking the cells of the kidney are now foreign "invaders," the body manufactures antibodies that attack and destroy the glomerular tissue—and with it the ability of the kidney to function.

> *The ability of mercury to incite autoimmune responses is likely due to the metal's capacity to bind to critical enzymes and proteins, thereby changing the structure of the proteins.*

Similar autoimmune-mediated damage occurs in the protective myelin sheaths of nerve cells and can be seen in multiple sclerosis, an autoimmune disease that causes various neuromuscular disorders. Destruction of the myelin sheath as a consequence of the binding of myelin proteins with mercury distorts their structure and provokes attack by the immune system T cells.[15,16]

Another autoimmune disease linked to mercury toxicity is lupus, which causes deterioration of the connective tissues, internal organs, bones and muscles. Rheumatoid arthritis, a chronic inflammation of the joints and connective tissues leading to painful disfigurement and loss of function, is also linked to mercury exposure.

The ability of mercury to incite autoimmune responses generally reflects the metal's capacity to bind to critical sulfur-containing enzymes and proteins, thereby changing the structure of these proteins and activating T cells to destroy them.[17] A 1994 Swedish study, in which mercury amalgam was implanted in the peritoneal cavities (the space within the abdominal cavity that contains the intestines and other organs) of mice, revealed an unsettling litany of immunosuppressive effects as well as evidence of a stimulatory autoimmune response.[18] Many researchers argue that mercury toxicity is, itself, an autoimmune disorder and that tests for mercury toxicity and assessment for amalgam removal should become a standard practice in the diagnosis of the constellation of symptoms that identify this disorder.[19]

NEUROLOGICAL

The CNS is the primary target for mercury vapor, and neurological problems are among the most common and most serious effects of mercury toxicity. Adverse behavioral effects due to low levels of exposure to mercury from amalgam fillings include the inability to make trivial decisions, resolve doubts, resist temptations and perform intellectual tasks.

Because the effects are so variable, mercury poisoning can be expressed as dementia, neurosis, psychosis, or simply dismissed as nervous "jitters." Today, we know that mercury from amalgams can cause or contribute to depression, schizophrenia, multiple sclerosis, erethism (abnormal irritability of cells or organs), amyotrophic lateral sclerosis (ALS) and Alzheimer's disease (AD).

Inactivation of Neurotransmitters

Acetylcholine (ACh) is an important neurotransmitter that transports nervous impulses across the synaptic gap, a tiny space separating nerve cells. Once the transferred signal has been received, ACh is broken down by the enzyme acetylcholinesterase (AChe). Mercury has been shown to elevate ACh,[20] which can lead to aggressive, violent and erratic behavior. Noradrenalin, an important excitatory neurotransmitter produced by the adrenal glands, is also influenced by mercury toxicity. The suppression of noradrenalin production deepens depressive states and increases mood disorders. *Serotonin*, an important mood enhancing neurotransmitter in the brain, is also suppressed with mercury exposure.

Such findings explain why, in a 1998 study conducted at Colorado State University, general health problems—particularly those related to mental and emotional health—were found to be 45 percent greater in those patients with amalgams.[21] Unexplained anger, irritability, anxiety and depression subsided or disappeared within one year after subjects had their dental amalgams removed.

Excitotoxicity

Astrocytes are a type of cell in the CNS that have the job of clearing metabolic debris from around nerve cells, modifying the ionic and amino acid concentrations, and regulating brain energy metabolism. Mercury dramatically diminishes astrocyte activity in the brain,[22] causing a toxic buildup of glutamate.[23,24] High levels of this neurotransmitter, in turn, cause excitotoxicity. Nerve cells in certain regions of the brain can become so overstimulated that they undergo a process of induced cell death, called *apoptosis*. It appears that the excess glutamate binds with receptors on the surfaces of nerve cells, causing a rapid inflow of calcium, which is lethal to the cell.

Increased intracellular calcium also contributes to the degradation of motor nerve function, observed in ALS. As well, glutamate-induced calcium aberrations contribute to the gradual extinction of brain cells in the hippocampus, a region of the brain responsible for recall and memory. Loss of these cells appears to be an underlying cause of AD.[25] Glutamate-induced neurotoxicity and related calcium toxicity, both a consequence of mercury exposure, appear to be principal factors in neural degeneration as seen in multiple sclerosis and Parkinson's disease.[26]

Disruption of Microtubules

One of mercury's most insidious effects stems from the metal's ability to disrupt the production of microtubules in brain cells.[27] These microskeletal-like structures, manufactured from tubulin proteins, are vital in the maintenance of proper cell structure. Recent work by Canadian researchers provides convincing visual evidence of mercury-induced disintegration of microtubules in brain cells. Loss of microtubule integrity, in turn, disrupts cell membrane structure and causes the formation of neurofibrillary tangles, so evident in Alzheimer's disease.[28] Similar observations are also reported in a Swiss study that showed nerve cells exposed to mercury increased their production of amyloid protein, which makes up the tangled plaques found in the autopsied brains of Alzheimer's patients.[29]

The Alzheimer's Connection: Research toxicologist, Dr. Boyd Haley, contends that having a mouthful of mercury from age 14 until age 65 and beyond greatly increases susceptibility to AD. Mercury easily penetrates the CNS and is one of the most notorious and aggressive inhibitors of sulfur-containing enzymes—the same enzymes whose inactivation is seen in AD. As well, the brains of autopsied AD patients exhibit mercury levels significantly higher than those who have died of other causes.[30] Flu shots, which contain both mercury and aluminum, have been found to increase the risk of AD by tenfold in those receiving multiple immunizations within a ten-year span.[31]

In a collaborative effort between Canadian and American researchers, laboratory rats were exposed to carefully controlled dosages of mercury, mimicking the levels normally found in the mouths of people with amalgam fillings. Their findings revealed that the rats quickly deteriorated and developed brain lesions identical to those found in autopsies of AD patients.[32] According to Dr. Haley, coauthor of the study, the results of the experiment were so disturbing he immediately resolved to get his fillings taken out and asked his wife to do the same.[33]

In summary, the very nature of mercury toxicity explains why those affected do not all react in the same manner or develop the same symptoms of disease. There is simply no predictable pattern to the onset of symptoms or to the level of individual sensitivity to the toxin. By

> *"Mercury should be considered as a causal contributor [to Alzheimer's disease] since the mercury can produce the two pathological hallmarks of the disease and inhibits the same thiol-sensitive enzymes that are dramatically inhibited in the AD brain."*
>
> — Dr. Boyd E Haley,
> Congressional testimony to the Committee on
> Government Reform, Washington DC, 2001

exploiting the weakest link in our defenses, mercury poisoning touches each of us in different ways—just how it will affect any one person we cannot be certain.

However, of this we *can* be certain: mercury is poisonous and if you are exposed to it for long enough your health is going to pay the price.

CHAPTER 9

Detoxification Mechanisms

"Diseases are crises of purification, of toxic elimination."
— Hippocrates,
circa 460-370 B.C.

Our ancestors had no reason to be concerned about mercury poisoning. Except for small amounts released from natural events, almost everyone lived an entire lifetime free from exposure to this toxic metal. Today, however, the average person's body contains between 10 to15 milligrams (mg) of mercury. Even without dental amalgams, it is extremely difficult to avoid exposure. No thanks to modern industry, mercury is now in our food, water, and even the air we breathe. It is added to fungicides and pesticides, cosmetics, and medicines—hundreds of products in all.

Fortunately, the human body has powerful detoxification systems to protect it from toxins such as mercury. Unfortunately, in today's world, the amount of toxic influences to which we are exposed continues to rise, and each year sees the addition of thousands of chemicals that have never before existed. Consequently, we need to assist the body in ridding itself of these toxic substances, especially mercury. The most effective way to do this is by supplementing the diet with compounds that can support the body's natural detoxification systems. In general, these compounds act in one of two phases of detoxification, and sometimes in both.

Phase One involves rendering the mercury more water-soluble; Phase Two involves binding the mercury to another molecule to form an excretable complex, which can then be removed from the body, primarily in the feces and the urine. Many of the nutrients that help protect the body from mercury toxicity are also potent antioxidants, so they provide additional health benefits.

Glutathione

For mercury detoxification, the most potent protectant manufactured by the body is glutathione (GSH), a small protein composed of three amino acids: glutamic acid, cysteine and glycine. GSH is a powerful antioxidant, a molecule that donates electrons to quench damaging free radicals. It is the chemical nature of the sulfur-containing amino acid, cysteine, that accounts for the antioxidant punch of GSH.

While GSH is found in every cell and in all the organs of the body, especially high amounts are found in the liver. So dependent is the body on the detoxifying action of GSH that intracellular glutathione status is a principal indicator of cellular health and of the cell's ability to resist toxic challenge.[1,2] Depletion of GSH can result in extensive damage to the mitochondria, where free radicals are generated as a side effect of the energy production process. In fact, depletion of mitochondrial GSH may be the ultimate factor determining a cell's vulnerability to oxidative attack.[3]

Within the specialized cells of the liver, GSH is conjugated (chemically joined) with solvents, fat-soluble pesticides, toxic chemicals, and other xenobiotics (materials foreign to the cell), such as mercury. Conjugation of a toxin with GSH renders the toxin water-soluble and prepares it for excretion from the body via the kidneys and the bile. The power of glutathione in the conjugation and elimination of toxins is prodigious. As the body's major cellular detoxification mechanism, GSH conjugation accounts for up to 60 percent of all liver metabolites in the bile.[4]

In fact, formation of the GSH-mercury complex is one of the few known mechanisms by which the body can flush the toxin back across the blood-brain barrier and out of brain tissue.[5] Astrocytes, the cells lining the blood-brain barrier that protect the CNS from toxins, are particularly rich in GSH; however, these GSH levels can easily be depleted. Consequently, enhancing astrocyte GSH stores has been found to markedly increase elimination of mercury from brain tissue.[6]

> *"The glutathione status of the cell...will perhaps turn out to be the most accurate indicator of the health of the cell. That is, as glutathione levels go, so will go the health of the cell."*
>
> —Dr. Parris Kidd

GSH binds to mercury in order to transport it out of the body. The binding and subsequent elimination of the mercury-GSH complex can rapidly diminish cellular GSH. For every atom of mercury that is eliminated, two molecules of GSH must be sacrificed. Once mercury is captured by GSH it cannot be released; therefore the body must expel the good with the bad. The consequence, of course, is the unavoidable loss of this vitally important antioxidant and cellular protector. Additional cellular GSH is lost as it performs its critically important role as a free-radical antagonist. This depletion of cellular GSH can only be made good through the remanufacture of the molecule by the cells or by replenishment through the consumption of foods rich in the precursors of GSH, particularly cysteine.

Depletion of cellular glutathione has consequences that go well beyond detoxification. Inadequate GSH levels may severely reduce immune functions,[7,8] thereby increasing vulnerability to infection.[9,10] Depletion of cellular GSH is also implicated in the development of several neurological disorders.[11] This comes as no surprise when we consider that the brain, highly oxygenated and rich in polyunsaturated lipids, is a fertile area for free-radical induced oxidative assault. Low GSH levels have been reported in Parkinson's[12] and Alzheimer's patients,[13] and it is probable that GSH depletion from a toxic overload of mercury plays a central role in the manifestation of these neurological diseases.

To summarize, with respect to the removal of mercury and other heavy metals, GSH plays three specific roles:

1. As a carrier, GSH binds aggressively with mercury, sacrificing itself to form a conjugated complex and thereby preventing the poison from damaging structural proteins and inactivating enzymes.

2. GSH-mercury complexes, once formed, are removed from tissues

and organs and eliminated from the body through the feces and urine.[14]

3. As a powerful free-radical scavenger, GSH increases the antioxidant status of the cell and defends against hydrogen peroxide and other free-radical species, including lipid peroxides produced by mercury.[15,16]

I believe that glutathione's greatest enemy is mercury. If the source of mercury contamination is not removed, glutathione levels will become depleted and the ability of the body to remove mercury will be seriously compromised. This will result in a slow but accelerating accumulation of mercury in the body that coincides with the abatement of GSH levels and the eventual development of chronic toxicity symptoms.

> *Glutathione's greatest enemy is mercury. If the source of contamination is not removed, glutathione levels will become depleted and the ability of the body to remove mercury will be seriously compromised.*

Nutrition for Detoxification

There are several nutrients that play an important role in mercury detoxification. Many of these participate in the glutathione peroxidase pathway, a vital antioxidant system of the cell that removes toxic hydrogen peroxide from the body. A study of patients with multiple sclerosis found that supplementation with high doses of selenium, vitamin C and vitamin E raised glutathione peroxidase (GSH-Px) activity five-fold, conferring a marked enhancement of cellular antioxidant status.[17] It stands to reason that such protection would offer significant benefit to anyone suffering from mercury poisoning. Other nutrients involved in the GSH-Px system are riboflavin (vitamin B_2) and niacin (vitamin B_3). Both nutrients are important for their role in the energy transfer reactions that are the driving force of this vital antioxidant enzyme system.

Several antioxidants, including vitamins A, C, E and beta-carotene (a precursor of vitamin A), and the mineral selenium, can also help reduce mercury toxicity by quenching the rampant free-radical generation that is a hallmark of the metal's presence. In addition, some of these nutrients have been found to provide further assistance in replenishing GSH levels.

In particular, supplementation with vitamin C has been found to enhance and maintain optimal tissue glutathione levels, provided the necessary metabolic precursors for glutathione synthesis are also available. One double-blind study found that red blood cell GSH levels increased nearly 50 percent when subjects were given 500 mg per day of ascorbic acid (vitamin C).[18] Vitamin C boosts GSH levels by helping the body manufacture it within the cells.

When given orally, such as through nutritional supplements, S-adenosyl methionine (SAM-e) is also effective in raising red blood cell and liver GSH.[19] Cysteine, the metabolic precursor that most severely limits the synthesis of glutathione, is another nutrient that has proven very effective in boosting GSH levels.[20] N-Acetyl Cysteine (NAC) is a precursor of cysteine; in the cell, NAC converts easily to cysteine, which, in turn, converts to GSH. NAC has been found to significantly boost GSH levels in deficient subjects.

The antioxidant alpha-lipoic acid (ALA) can penetrate the blood-brain barrier to reach and bind with inorganic mercury trapped within the CNS.[21] Supplementation with ALA also enhances cellular and extra-cellular levels of GSH;[22] in animal studies it has been shown to dramatically increase the release of inorganic mercury by stimulating the release of GSH into the bile.[23]

The GSH-mediated removal process goes on every day; consequently, unless the body's glutathione stores are constantly replenished, a serious depletion of GSH will occur. Supplementation with these nutrients can make a substantial difference in the body's cellular GSH status and its ability to handle mercury and other heavy metals.

Table 9-1

Nutrients Involved in Glutathione Metabolism

Nutrient	Effects on Glutathione Status
Vitamin C	Antioxidant, maintains tissue GSH levels
Beta-Carotene	Antioxidant, enhances GSH production
Vitamin E	Antioxidant, enhances GSH production
Selenium	Antioxidant mineral, GSH cofactor
N-Acetyl-Cysteine	GSH precursor; raises GSH levels
Alpha-Lipoic Acid	Chelator; enhances cellular and extracellular GSH
SAM-e	Raises RBC and liver GSH levels
Riboflavin	Facilitates GSH-Px system
Niacin	Facilitates GSH-Px system
Cysteine	Metabolic precursor; raises GSH levels

MEASURING MERCURY IN THE BODY

Most investigators use blood and urine levels of mercury to determine toxicity; however, these are not the tests of choice to assess how well your body is removing mercury. Up to 90 percent of the mercury removed naturally by the body is expelled via the feces; therefore, the fecal-metals test can provide a much clearer picture of how much mercury your body removes on a daily basis.

If, through the fortunes of a healthy diet and the wisdom of supplementation, a person's nutritional status is optimized, that individual will exhibit a marked tolerance toward mercury.

The fecal-metals test reveals that a person with amalgam fillings generally excretes much higher levels of mercury than a person who does not have amalgam fillings. This, in turn, reflects a higher body burden of the poison. Physicians regard this test as an accurate and important way to measure body levels of mercury and other heavy metals.

In summary, it is likely that the wide range of symptoms associated with chronic mercury poisoning within a given population has much to do with the nutritional status of the individual. We know that mercury exerts its presence as a powerful oxidizing agent and a prodigious inhibitor of enzymes; however, mercury must first overcome the defenses of several protective antioxidants, including vitamins A, C, E, B_2, B_3, beta-carotene, the antioxidant mineral selenium, alpha-lipoic acid, N-acetyl cysteine and GSH.[24]

Through a healthy diet and the wisdom of supplementation, individuals whose nutritional status is optimized will exhibit a marked tolerance toward mercury. This does not make the mercury any less poisonous, but it does mean that the body is better able to protect itself from the metal's toxic effects. While these measures cannot, by themselves, fully protect against a sustained toxic challenge, the level of risk for those individuals will be appreciably lowered. On the other hand, individuals whose inadequate diets and unhealthy lifestyles already place them under undue oxidative stress will be much more vulnerable to the toxic consequences of long-term mercury exposure.

Unfortunately, most North Americans—adults and children alike—fall within the latter category.

CHAPTER 10

The Dental Office— A Hazardous Workplace

"There is nothing more toxic in a dentist's office than mercury—unless you have some plutonium lying around."[1]
—Charles Brown,
Consumers for Dental Choice

Professor Lars Friberg, a distinguished toxicologist and expert advisor on heavy-metal toxicity to WHO, states that mercury should be regarded as a chemical carcinogen. He also emphasizes that there is no safe level of exposure.[2]

In the past, the conventional view has been that if mercury presented a significant hazard, its effects would have surfaced long ago. We now understand, however, that mercury poisoning is cumulative and that disease symptoms may not show up for years and perhaps decades after a person is first exposed.

LEVELS OF OCCUPATIONAL EXPOSURE

Dentists and dental personnel who have worked with amalgam restorations over long periods of time are found to have significant levels of mercury in their bodies. Momentary and repeated exposure to high levels of mercury during insertion, polishing, and removal of amalgams—particularly if adequate preventive measures are not taken—can add substantially to the body burden of dental personnel. A 1985 study reports mercury concentrations approaching 1,000 µg/m^3 in the breathing zone of dentists not using adequate coolant or aspiration techniques during operative procedures.[3]

Mercury levels in the urine of dental personnel average about two times those of the general population. Older dentists exhibit urine mercury levels about four times that of nondental professionals, and have significantly elevated brain mercury levels. Autopsies conducted on elderly dentists have found mercury levels in some parts of the brain as much as 80 times higher than normal.[4]

The accumulated body burden of mercury in dental personnel has been shown to reach ten times the levels of nonoccupationally exposed (control) individuals.[5-7] Dentists also have elevated skeletal mercury levels, demonstrate a propensity for mercury retention, and exhibit mercury levels in their hair and nails 50 to 300 percent higher than controls.

Given that most dental offices have atmospheric mercury levels that far exceed U.S. guidelines for safety, it is not surprising to find that many dentists suffer from mercury poisoning. According to one study, the impact of occupational exposure on urinary mercury levels in dental personnel corresponds to that released by 19 amalgam fillings.[8] Atmospheric levels of mercury in dental offices have been found be as high as 300 µg/m^3.[9] In fact, in Canada and the U.S. the level of mercury vapor in most dental offices is considerably above the guidelines set by Health Canada, the U.S. EPA and the U.S. ATSDR.[10] According to this information, dental offices are certainly hazardous worksites!

High brain levels of mercury are also confirmed in autopsies of former dental workers, who exhibit ten-fold elevations in the pituitary gland, along with significantly elevated levels in other regions of the brain. One study, conducted by Swedish researchers, found that concentrations of mercury in the pituitaries of deceased dental workers were 35 times that of the normal population.[11]

The WHO reports similar findings on occupational exposure, including dental personnel. Autopsy data showed high mercury concentrations in the brain years after cessation of exposure, indicating that once mercury is deposited in the brain it takes up long-term residence. Among deceased dental staff, mercury levels reached milligram-per-kilogram levels within the pituitary tissue, demonstrating the metal's propensity to accumulate at extraordinarily high levels in the body's master gland.[12]

> *In Canada and the U.S. the level of mercury vapor in most dental offices is considerably above the guidelines set by Health Canada, the U.S. EPA and the U.S. ATSDR. According to this information, dental offices are certainly hazardous worksites!*

Urine mercury levels in dental personnel are highly correlated with the number of amalgams placed or restored during the week, the number of amalgams polished during the week, and the number of amalgams resident in the mouth of the individual dental professional. Moreover, both the dental hygienist and the patient have been found to receive high doses of mercury when an ultrasonic scaler is used or amalgam surfaces are polished. As well, the use of a high-speed drill in removal or replacement of amalgams creates a high volume of mercury vapor, along with particulate matter and airborne dust, which is rapidly absorbed into the oral mucosa and lungs. Even when precautions are used, such as a dental dam, dental mask and aspiration, both patient and practitioner can absorb considerable dust and mercury vapor, which moves rapidly into the blood.

Effects of Occupational Exposure

Researchers have identified significant deficits in muscle control and peripheral nerve function amongst dental personnel who were occupationally exposed to elemental mercury and its vapor. Such deficits have been statistically correlated to the body burden of mercury in these individuals. Dental personnel exhibit considerably greater neurological, memory, mood and behavioral problems, which appear to increase in severity with the years of occupational exposure.[13]

One study, conducted by the Occupational Health and Safety Program of the Harvard School of Public Health, found significantly elevated suicide rates among dentists, compared to other college-educated professionals. A similar South African study found that ten percent of dentists suffered from severe suicidal intention.[14] While neither of these studies can suggest cause and effect, the findings are indicative of the numerous neurological symptoms of mercury toxicity reported elsewhere and point to the need for further investigation of the mental-health consequences of mercury exposure.

Simply put, dentists have the highest suicide rate of any profession, along with an inordinately high incidence of depression, memory and emotional disorders—mercury may well be the culprit.

> *Dentists have the highest suicide rate of any profession and an inordinately high incidence of depression, memory and emotional disorders.*

In a 1998 study on the neurobehavioral effects of mercury exposure in dental personnel, researchers found convincing evidence of adverse behavioral effects, even at low exposures within the range experienced by the general population.[15] Along with chronic fatigue, likely due to toxic overload, dental personnel also frequently suffer from chronic pain, an inability to concentrate, and impaired neurobehavioral skills such as muscle response, visual motor coordination, memory, and reaction to stress factors.

The Female Practitioner/Hygienist

For the female practitioner, the consequences of occupationally related mercury toxicity are even more alarming. Epidemiological evidence reveals that women who work in dental offices have increased rates of spontaneous abortions and breast pathologies that are directly related to the length of time on the job.[16] Rowland and coworkers found that the probability of female dental assistants conceiving was 63 percent less than women who were not occupationally exposed to mercury.[17]

Female technicians who work with mercury amalgam have also been found to have increased menstrual difficulties, reduced fertility, a lowered probability of conception, and increased spontaneous abortions, a finding which has also been observed in the wives of workers occupationally exposed to high levels of mercury.[18] In addition, the offspring of female technicians are at greater risk of having a congenital deformity and have a lower IQ, compared to the normal population.[19]

Dental practitioners working in an environment where amalgams are placed or restored must consider carefully the consequences of long-term mercury exposure. With the availability of biocompatible composites to replace mercury amalgam, the continued use of this poisonous material poses a needless and unacceptable health risk to practitioners, staff and patients.

CHAPTER 11

Variations in Mercury Exposure

"I don't want to panic people, but I think we have to be realistic. Mercury comes out of amalgams. It gets into our saliva, and we swallow it. The vapors go through the membranes of our mouth to the nasal mucosa and collect in the brain."

—Dr. Boyd Haley,
University of Kentucky

In the world of pharmaceuticals, every drug has benefits and risks, and health professionals take this into account when prescribing a product for patient use. If the benefits for the patient clearly outweigh the risks, the drug has therapeutic value; if the risks far outweigh the benefits, the drug should not be used. Moreover, in prescribing a particular drug, the physician considers the patient's general health, potential for allergic reaction, body size and any other mitigating factors. Even when a drug has merit, a physician will not give the same dosage to everyone.

For good reason, pharmaceutical manufacturers list the prescribed therapeutic dosage of a drug in micrograms, milligrams, or grams per kilogram of body weight, as well as specific contraindications for use. Baby aspirin, for example, allows an analgesic dosage appropriate to a very small body weight; the dosage for an adult would, necessarily, be different. As well, a vast number of prescribed drugs are contraindicated for pregnant or nursing women because of unacceptable risks for the developing fetus. Adjustment of dosage and attention to specified contraindications for a pharmaceutical product is sound medical guidance and the best means of minimizing undesired—even fatal—side effects.

The fact that physicians take individual differences into account when prescribing a potentially toxic drug would lead one to expect that dentists would do the same when placing poisonous amalgam fillings into a patient's mouth. A careful assessment of a patient's sensitivity to mercury, current body burden, length of exposure to previous amalgam fillings, biological age, risk of pregnancy, and an evaluation of behavioral patterns that stimulate excessive release of mercury, would seem prudent measures to take.

Most dentists don't do *any* of this. It matters not whether you are sensitive to mercury, already have a mouthful of metal, or are experiencing mercury-related disease symptoms. It matters not whether you have been exposed to mercury since conception or you are planning to become or are already pregnant—to most conventional dentists a cavity is a cavity and the most profitable way to fill it is to plug it with mercury amalgam. End of story.

A FORGOTTEN DOCTRINE

When it comes to the use of mercury fillings by conventional dentists, the Hippocratic Oath of "First, do no harm," venerated by physicians, appears to be a long-forgotten doctrine. Despite the wealth of scientific evidence that now prevails, the ADA remains adamant that, no matter how much mercury your amalgam fillings release, they are harmless. A seven-year-old child could have the same number and size of fillings as a grown adult and, as a result, absorb just as much mercury. According to the ADA, this issue is irrelevant.

Largely because of the ADA's continued denial that mercury amalgam is harmful, most dentists use it in their practice without consideration of contraindications for use. In keeping with this stance, the ADA has not developed any guidelines for evaluation of allergic responses, adjustments for length of previous exposure, consideration of current body burden, or correlation of weight and dosage. Nor has the Association identified any precautions regarding fetal toxicity.

> *When it comes to the use of mercury fillings by conventional dentists, the Hippocratic Oath of "First, do no harm," appears a long-forgotten doctrine.*

After all, why bother? To do so would be to admit that mercury is a poison and that, collectively, the dental profession, specifically the ADA and most conventional dentists, has been woefully remiss in protecting the health of the patient. Tragically, this position shows total disregard for public health and safety—it is also a position that may prove costly should future legal actions be launched.

SOURCES OF EXPOSURE

To determine an individual's level of exposure to mercury released by amalgams, two general sources of exposure must be considered: the first relates to mercury exposure as a consequence of dental treatment; the second relates to how the fillings are stimulated after they have been placed in your teeth.

Mercury Exposure During Dental Treatment

This category of exposure includes placement process, removal protocol, number and size of the fillings, and composition of the amalgam, among others. While everyone should be concerned about this, it is the woman who is pregnant, nursing, or planning to have children who should be particularly vigilant. I strongly recommend that women never have amalgam fillings placed or removed while pregnant or nursing.

Placement Process

When the pliable mercury amalgam mixture is placed in the cavity, it is compressed and then carved to fit the shape of the tooth. This process releases significant amounts of particulate amalgam and mercury vapor.

In fact, the greatest dental exposure to elemental mercury vapor occurs when an amalgam filling is placed or removed. The amount that is released during the placement procedure can be measured in milligrams—thousands of micrograms—per cubic meter of air. This is far higher than the amount of mercury a filling will release after it has hardened, regardless of how it is stimulated.

During placement, particularly if a dental dam is not used, the patient unavoidably swallows elemental mercury and amalgam particles. Bacteria in the mouth and intestine, which have the ability to rapidly transform elemental mercury into organic mercury, swing into action and produce the more toxic methylmercury, which is then readily absorbed into the body. This large and acute exposure to mercury creates a potential crisis for those who are allergic to the toxin. As well, if the patient is pregnant or nursing, it poses a substantial health risk to the fetus or nursing child. Anyone with an existing health issue, especially a compromised immune system, is also exceedingly vulnerable to this toxic burden.

I believe that "mercury shock," characterized by symptoms of a nonfatal acute dose of elemental mercury, accounts for many of the effects people experience after the placement of amalgam fillings. Symptoms include headaches, coughing, sore gums, chest pain, nausea, diarrhea, and difficulty with breathing. Depending on the level of exposure, post-operative reactions could also include fine tremors in the fingers, toes, eyelids, lips and tongue; insomnia; irritability; transient personality changes; abnormal response to stimulation; and memory loss. Other common nonspecific symptoms include exhaustion, visual problems, mental fogginess, speech problems, and difficulty with balance while walking.

Led to believe that mercury amalgams are perfectly safe, most people do not associate any of these symptoms with the placement of their fillings. Too frequently, patients will dismiss their symptoms as a mere consequence of an exhaustive and traumatic dental appointment. To complicate matters, most often the acute symptoms will subside; consequently, people who experience them seldom "connect the dots" to the dental visit. If they do seek treatment for any of the postoperative symptoms, it will likely be with a health professional and not with their dentist. As a result, the issue of mercury poisoning may never be linked to the symptoms presented during a medical diagnosis.

Removal Protocol

Unless a safe amalgam-removal protocol is followed, the extraction of mercury amalgam results in the second-greatest exposure to mercury. The traditional removal procedure is to drill out the fillings, which generates a great deal of heat and dramatically increases the release of mercury vapor. It also releases amalgam particles, which are subsequently swallowed.

The same symptomatic reactions associated with placement of fillings can be observed with their removal. The number of fillings removed, sensitivity to mercury, and the general health of the individual determine the extent of these effects. In many dental offices, it is a common procedure for several older or broken amalgam fillings to be removed and replaced with new amalgam fillings during the same appointment. This, of course, will radically increase exposure to mercury.

> *Led to believe that mercury amalgams are perfectly safe, most people don't associate any of these symptoms with the placement of fillings.*

Number and Size of Fillings

The more amalgam fillings that you have in your teeth, the greater will be your exposure to mercury and to the risk of developing symptoms and diseases related to chronic mercury toxicity. Amalgam fillings are generally classified by the number of surfaces they contain and these variations in size will have a significant effect on the extent of mercury exposure. For example, all else being the same, brushing two small amalgams releases more mercury than brushing one small amalgam.

The average adult American has ten amalgam fillings, each containing an average of three surfaces, with each surface releasing approximately one microgram of mercury per day.[1] This means that the average adult exposure equals 30 micrograms of elemental mercury per day, more than tenfold above the cautionary limit for mercury exposure from food, issued by the U.S. Food and Drug Administration. According to the Toxic Element Research Foundation (TERF), people with 13 or more amalgam fillings can exceed the daily mercury exposure limit of 42.9 micrograms issued by the World Health Organization.[2] It is compelling to note that the TERF data do not include mercury exposure from other non-amalgam sources—if it had, the level of exposure would have been even greater.

Composition of the Amalgam

As the following table demonstrates, the proportions of the various materials used to produce an amalgam filling vary, depending on the manufacturer. While mercury is, by far, the most poisonous metal in amalgam, tin and silver can also be toxic or allergenic.

Table 11-1

Composition of Dental Amalgam

Mercury	48 - 60%
Silver	15 - 37%
Tin	12 - 13%
Copper	0 - 26%
Zinc	0 - 1%

With a mercury content averaging 56 percent by weight, a new amalgam filling can contain from 500,000 to 1,000,000 micrograms of elemental mercury, depending on its size. However, as fillings age they lose a considerable amount of mercury. Many studies have shown that the mercury content of five- to ten-year-old fillings is reduced to only 25 to 30 percent of the initial amount.[3] Consequently, over the estimated ten-year lifespan of an amalgam filling, up to 50 percent of the mercury—250,000 to 500,000 micrograms—will be released. The good news is that there is less mercury in the filling to be released; the bad news is that up to 87 percent of the "lost" mercury has been absorbed into the body.

Type of Amalgam Filling

Around 1990, dentists began replacing the traditional amalgam material with the nongamma-2 amalgam material, which contains more copper. The new amalgam mixture was created to reduce oxidation of the filling surface and make it more resistant to fractures. However, the addition of copper did far more than make the filling stronger: it also generated a greater galvanic current, a common occurrence when two or more metals of differing electrochemical potentials are brought into contact. Unfortunately, the reduced oxide layer in combination with the stronger galvanic current of the nongamma-2 amalgams actually causes droplets of mercury to form on the surface of the fillings when they are subjected to stimulation, such as chewing and brushing.[4] This results in a release of mercury that is up to 50 times greater than that of the older amalgams.

This so-called "improvement" in the new amalgam material may help its strength and aesthetics, but it comes at a substantially greater risk to your health. For this reason, the continued use of non-gamma-2 amalgam makes no sense and only serves to highlight the total disregard by the dental industry toward the doctrine of "First, do no harm."

Age of Amalgam Fillings

The amount of mercury you are exposed to from your amalgam fillings also relates to how long they have been in your teeth. Someone who has had amalgam fillings for only a few months will not have been exposed to the same amount of mercury as someone who has had them for years. Mercury toxicity is a form of retention toxicity; consequently, your total body burden of mercury will reflect not only the number and size of your amalgam fillings but also how long you have had them. The longer the fillings have been in your teeth, the more mercury has been deposited in your body and the greater will be its toxic effect on all body functions.

Cleaning and Polishing

Use of the *Cavitron®* or any other ultrasonic tooth cleaner on the surfaces of amalgam fillings can rapidly heat the fillings and increase the release of mercury vapor. Some dentists polish amalgams shortly after placing them to make them shiny and extend the life of the filling. This exposes the patient to extremely high levels of mercury vapor during, and for some time after, polishing. In fact, polishing the surfaces of amalgam fillings will also release amalgam particles that contain mercury (which are then swallowed or converted in the saliva to methylmercury) and can generate mercury vapor levels as high as 4200 $\mu g/m^3$.

> *If your amalgam fillings are shiny and have a bright*
> *silver color, they have been polished- and you have been*
> *exposed to exceedingly high levels of mercury.*

If your amalgam fillings are shiny and have a bright silver color, they have been polished—and you have been exposed to exceedingly high levels of mercury vapor. If you were not advised of this before you consented to a dental polish, you should have been.

Mercury Exposure through Amalgam Stimulation

A variety of factors conspire to influence the amount of mercury released from amalgam fillings. While the dental industry continues to deny it, whenever you do anything that stimulates your amalgams, mercury vapor is released and absorbed through the lungs and oral mucosa and passes into the body. During active stimulation, and for as long as 90 minutes after, mercury vapor levels in the mouth can exceed the limits of safety set by some regulatory agencies. Remember that each surface of a dental filling releases approximately one microgram of mercury per day.[5] Also remember that up to 87 percent of the mercury vapor released from an amalgam enters the body, and a significant portion of this passes directly to the brain, where it is retained for decades.

To determine the total amount of mercury exposure, one must consider the several avenues whereby oral stimulation can increase the amount of mercury released by amalgam fillings. The following categories provide information on ways that you can unintentionally increase the release of mercury from amalgam fillings:

Chewing

Chewing releases mercury from your fillings. Researchers evaluating the mercury content of the expired air of subjects with amalgams found a 16-fold increase after chewing, while the expired air of the nonamalgam group remained unchanged.[6] While all forms of eating can trigger the release of mercury, some foods have a greater effect than others. Abrasive foods (such as nuts and seeds) disrupt the protective oxide layer, heat, and abrade the fillings through friction, thereby releasing significant amounts of mercury vapor and amalgam particles into the oral cavity. Snacking also increases the release of mercury vapor, as does eating acidic foods. Acidic fruit juices and soft drinks can also trigger the release of mercury vapor by etching the surfaces of amalgam fillings.

In a 1985 study conducted at the University of Calgary, researchers found that subjects with amalgams who chewed gum for ten minutes released about six times more mercury vapor when chewing than when at rest. The release of mercury from dental amalgams by oral stimulation exceeds a major percentage of internationally accepted limits and plays a major role in the total daily dosage of mercury absorbed by individuals.[7]

And the more you chew, the worse it gets. Compulsive gum chewing can increase the intraoral levels of mercury concentration up to 54 times that of unstimulated fillings.[8] Therefore, a person who only has a few amalgam fillings but is a serious gum chewer releases far more mercury each day than a person with a mouthful of mercury who doesn't chew gum.

Brushing

The simple act of brushing your teeth can substantially increase the release of mercury into the oral cavity.[9] How hard, how long, and how often the teeth are brushed influences the amount of mercury released. Brushing with a hard toothbrush and abrasive toothpaste can increase mercury vapor levels in the mouth to as high as 272 $\mu g/m^3$.[10]

Using an electric toothbrush releases more mercury vapor than a manual toothbrush. Although some people use an electric toothbrush for a shorter period of time, the total amount of mercury released can still be significantly higher than from manual brushing.

Many dentists recommend dry brushing, which means brushing with no toothpaste. Dry brushing greatly increases the release of mercury vapor because toothpaste absorbs some of the mercury vapor that amalgam fillings release when they are brushed.

Bruxism

Up to 90 percent of the U.S. population grind their teeth, a habitual characteristic known as bruxism. Bruxism disrupts the oxide layer and, through friction, appreciably heats the filling. In most cases, bruxism significantly increases the release of mercury vapor from amalgam fillings.

This habit is particularly harmful because most tooth grinders do much of their work at night. Consequently, this unconscious action may occur for eight or more hours in a 24-hour period, continuously exposing the body to high levels of mercury during this time. Like gum chewers, a tooth grinder with only a few amalgams can release considerably more mercury than a person who has more amalgams but is not a tooth grinder.

Galvanic Current

If a noble-metal filling, such as gold, is next to an amalgam filling, an electrical current flows between them (a noble metal is one that resists oxidation and dissolution by acids: gold, platinum, and silver are examples of noble metals). This galvanic current, caused by the differing electrochemical potentials of the metals, can markedly increase the release of mercury from amalgams. While a normal amalgam surface has been found to release about one microgram of mercury per day, galvanic induction can release from three to 1,000 micrograms of mercury per day.[11]

> *Tissue levels of mercury near a gold cap on an amalgam filling can easily reach an astounding 1,000 ppm (1,000 mg/kg) due to the galvanic action between gold and amalgam.*

The average mercury levels in tissue next to mercury fillings is about 200 parts per million (ppm), or 200 mg/kg of tissue; however, levels near a gold cap on an amalgam filling can easily reach an astounding 1,000 ppm (1,000 mg/kg) due to the galvanic action between the gold and the amalgam.[12]

In one case, German oral surgeons found a mercury level in the jaw bone under gold crowns placed over amalgams that exceeded 5,760 ppm.[13] This is one of the highest levels of mercury contamination ever measured in living tissues and is magnitudes higher than the one-ppm limit for the prohibition of foods, issued by the FDA.

Galvanic action occurs 24 hours a day and is not related to any other form of stimulation. Health Canada and several other government agencies now advise against the use of mixed metals, such as gold and amalgams; however, many practitioners ignore these warnings.

Other Amalgam Stimulants

Bathing and taking saunas can increase the release of mercury. Hot baths and saunas have great value, but they can increase the temperature of the oral cavity. The higher the temperature of the mouth, the more mercury is released.

The consumption of hot liquids and foods can increase the release of mercury up to 200 times that of an unstimulated amalgam. The amount of mercury released through the daily consumption of hot coffee and other beverages can add substantially to the total body burden.

Smoking increases the temperature in the mouth; it also increases the exposure to cadmium, another extremely toxic heavy metal that is believed to enhance the toxic effect of mercury.

WHERE DO YOU STAND?

You now have a clear picture of all the ways by which you can stimulate your amalgam fillings to release mercury. You also understand that each of these forms of stimulation increases your risk of exposure to this toxin.

The good news is that if you still have amalgam fillings in your teeth, there are a number of things you can do to reduce the amount of mercury to which you are being exposed—at least until you can have these toxic waste repositories removed for good! How to do this will be discussed in a later chapter.

After what you have read so far, how would you classify yourself with regard to your exposure to mercury from amalgam fillings? Would you say that you belong in a low-, medium-, or high-risk category—or are you just not sure?

I think it is time you found out.

CHAPTER 12

Assessing Your Mercury Risk

"The true impact of amalgam poisoning is similar to that of the Chernobyl tragedy. The magnitude of the crisis is not the few who have died from massive exposure, but rather the millions whose health will be eroded by the ongoing, small-dose poisoning."
— Toxic Element Research Foundation.

Despite the fact that over 150 million Americans have amalgam fillings, there are no existing standards for determining the level of risk from chronic mercury exposure. Consequently, this chapter includes a mercury risk assessment to address this inadequacy and assist individuals in evaluating their present level of risk. The *Mercury Risk Assessment* consists of a self-evaluation questionnaire that will place you in one of three risk categories: low, moderate, or high. By completing the following self-evaluation, you will discover where you currently are along the risk spectrum with regard to the hazard posed by your fillings and other sources of mercury exposure.

> We know that everyone with amalgam fillings accumulates mercury. We also know that the more mercury the body is exposed to, the more it retains.

Keep in mind that this self-evaluation is only a snapshot in time. It reflects your risk status at the time the evaluation was completed. Mercury toxicity is a form of retention toxicity and therefore is cumulative in nature. Consequently, the risk assessment score you receive when you complete this evaluation will worsen progressively over time—as long as your amalgam fillings remain in place.

Remember, mercury can never be broken down into a less toxic substance—mercury will always be mercury and must be removed from the body before any improvement in related health problems will be experienced.

The Risk Categories

There are three different categories of risk to mercury exposure: low, moderate, and high. While there are no precise dividing lines, the *Mercury Risk Assessment* can help you determine which category you are currently in.

Low Risk

Some people have no or very few amalgam fillings, received little or no mercury as a fetus or nursing child, and have no other contributing health concerns. These individuals are the fortunate ones who can be considered low risk.

If people in this category take care of themselves nutritionally, they may never manifest serious symptoms of chronic mercury poisoning. However, for those who have even a few amalgams, their detoxification systems will be under stress as long as these fillings are in place, and it is unlikely they will achieve optimal health. Over the years, the mercury released by their amalgam fillings will likely accumulate and may contribute to so-called "age-related" symptoms and illnesses.

If your fillings are properly removed and replaced while you are still in this category, you will have little accumulated mercury to remove and little damage to correct. Also, you will not have to participate in a mercury detoxification program that would be required if you were in the moderate- or high-risk category. If you are over 50 and have not exhibited any mercury-related symptoms, once you remove your existing fillings it is unlikely you will ever demonstrate observable signs of mercury toxicity.

Moderate Risk

People at moderate risk include those who have more amalgam fillings than in the low-risk category and those who have been exposed to more mercury from their mothers' amalgam fillings. It includes people who stimulate their fillings more intensely than those in the low-risk category. Also, it includes those who have had their fillings in place longer than those in the low-risk category. While the majority of people in the lower end of this category may not have developed a mercury-related disease, they will tend to exhibit more symptoms of mercury toxicity than people in the low-risk category.

If you fit into this category, consider the following: if you are under 40 and are already at the middle to high end of the moderate-risk category, there is a strong probability that you will develop one or more mercury-related diseases. You have many more years to accumulate mercury; consequently, there is some urgency in taking the necessary steps toward amalgam removal and mercury detoxification.

High Risk

Individuals in this category will have a substantial number of mercury risk factors and may already exhibit many of the more serious symptoms of mercury poisoning. The majority of people in this category will have had their fillings in place for a longer period of time and may have had greater exposure to other sources of mercury than those in the low- and medium-risk categories. Many individuals in this category were exposed to substantial amounts of mercury as a fetus and nursing child, and they likely received all or most of their vaccinations, thus adding substantially to their total body burden of mercury. Individuals in this category will also have been exposed to environmental sources of mercury, either through their occupation, their diet, or their proximity to a source of environmental release, such as a coal-fired power plant.

These individuals will have existing health issues and already may have developed one or more of the diseases associated with mercury poisoning. Chronic mercury poisoning may have also weakened their defense systems to the point where their bodies are vulnerable to other diseases, particularly those degenerative diseases related to oxidative stress from free radicals. In all probability, their overall health has been compromised and immediate medical intervention may be necessary. People in this category cannot afford to wait; immediate amalgam removal is warranted and participation in an aggressive detoxification program is essential.

The Mercury Risk Assessment

I invite you to take the following mercury risk assessment, developed by Dr. Tom McGuire. Keep in mind that this is not a rigorous clinical evaluation. The point system is only meant to give you a general idea of your risk category. The assessment is based on a number of common risk factors, and the rating for each category is weighted to reflect the amount of mercury released for each situation. You will be evaluated for eight different categories of mercury exposure:

- Amalgam Risk Factors
- Behavioral Risk Factors;
- General Risk Factors;
- Mercury-related Symptoms;
- Mercury-related Diseases;
- Other Debilitating Diseases;
- Occupation and Product Risks; and
- Environmental Exposure.

At the end of the assessment, a section is provided to record the accrued points for each category. Once you have assessed yourself in a single category, simply enter the total score for that category in the appropriate section in Table 12-4, at the end of the survey.

Some questions may be difficult to answer. For example, you may not know whether your mother had amalgam fillings when you were conceived and nursed. Also, you may not know how many vaccinations you received as a child. Because most people alive today had most of their vaccinations, I recommend answering **Yes** and circling the appropriate score. If you are under 60 years of age and do not know if your mother had amalgam fillings when you were conceived or nursed, I suggest answering **Yes** and circling the appropriate score. If you are over 60 and don't know, I suggest answering **No**, as it is less likely that your mother had amalgams at the time of your birth. Even without exact information, you can acquire a fairly accurate estimate of your mercury risk level.

While you should be able to complete the risk assessment on your own, you may wish to check with your dentist regarding tooth grinding and the number of amalgam fillings you currently have.

When you have finished scoring yourself in all risk categories, complete the calculation at the bottom of Table 12-4, and then compare *Total Risk* score to the *Risk Categories* scores in Table 12-5, at the end of this survey. This will provide you with your relative risk for exposure to mercury and will furnish guidance on the urgency of your decision regarding amalgam removal and participation in a mercury detoxification program. If your assessment places you in the moderate- to high-risk category, I strongly recommend a fecal-metals test to objectively confirm the assessment. Even if you fall into the low-risk category, if you experience any of the symptoms or diseases identified in the assessment, you may wish to consult with your health care provider regarding the fecal-metals test.

This evaluation is intended primarily for those individuals who currently have amalgam fillings; however, it will also provide useful information on exposure risks for those individuals who do not have amalgams. Please note that, because it is very difficult to verify a mercury allergy without a complete clinical evaluation, this assessment does not consider allergy to mercury as a risk factor.

PART I: Amalgam Risk Factors

1. Using the following scale, how many amalgam fillings do you currently have? Circle the appropriate score below your category.

No amalgams	1-4	5-8	9+
0	1	1.5	2

This is your *Amalgam Filling Score*. Please place your score in Section A of Table 12-4, at the end of this assessment.

If you do not have any amalgam fillings or have had them removed, please enter a score of 0 for your *Amalgam Filling Score*, your *Time Factor Score* and your *Personal Risk Factors score*, in Sections A, B and C of Table 12-4, at the end of this assessment.

If you have one or more amalgam fillings, PLEASE PROCEED TO QUESTION 2.

If you do not have amalgam fillings or have had them removed, PLEASE SKIP TO QUESTION 17. DO NOT COMPLETE QUESTIONS 2 TO 16.

Questions 2 to 16 are to be completed *only* by those respondents who have one or more amalgam fillings.

2. How many years has it been since you first had amalgam fillings? Circle the appropriate score below your category.

Less than 1 year	1-4	5-8	9 or more years
0	1.2	1.4	1.6

This is your Time Factor Score. Please place this score in Section B of Table 12-4, at the end of this assessment. Please proceed to the next questions.

PART II: Personal Risk Factors

3. Where "frequently" means several times a day, how often do you grind your teeth? Circle the appropriate score.

Never	Seldom	Sometimes	Frequently
0	10	20	30

4. Where "frequently" means several times a day, how often do you clench you teeth? Circle the appropriate score.

Never	Seldom	Sometimes	Frequently
0	10	20	30

5. Where "frequently" means several times a day, how often do you chew gum? Circle the appropriate score.

Never	Seldom	Sometimes	Frequently
0	10	20	30

6. Do you have both gold and amalgam fillings? Circle the appropriate score.

No	Yes
0	30

7. On average, how many meals do you normally eat in a day? Circle the appropriate score.

1 or less	2	3 or more
5	10	15

8. Where "frequently" means several times a day, how often do you snack between meals? Circle the appropriate score.

Never	Seldom	Sometimes	Frequently
0	5	10	15

9. On average, how many times a day do brush your teeth? Circle the appropriate score.

1 or less	2	3 or more
5	10	15

10. Where "frequently" means several times a day, how often do you use an electric tooth brush? Circle the appropriate score.

Never	Seldom	Sometimes	Frequently
0	5	10	15

11. Where "frequently" means several times a day, how frequently do you drink hot liquids? Circle the appropriate score.

Never	Seldom	Sometimes	Frequently
0	5	10	15

12. Where "frequently" means several times a day, how often do you eat abrasive foods, such as nuts or crunchy cereals? Circle the appropriate score.

Never	Seldom	Sometimes	Frequently
0	5	10	15

13. Where "frequently" means several times a day, how often do you drink acidic liquids, such as orange, tomato, pineapple juice or soda pop? Circle the appropriate score.

Never	Seldom	Sometimes	Frequently
0	5	10	15

14. Where "frequently" means several times a day, how often do you find yourself breathing through your mouth? Circle the appropriate score.

Never	Seldom	Sometimes	Frequently
0	5	10	15

15. Where "frequently" means several times a day, how often do you smoke? Circle the appropriate score.

Never	Seldom	Sometimes	Frequently
0	5	10	15

16. On a *weekly* basis, how often do you use a sauna, hot tub, or take hot baths? Circle the appropriate score.

Less than once/week	1-3 times/week	4-6 times/week	Daily
0	5	10	15

17. Questions 3 to 16 are your *Personal Risk Factor* scores. Please add up the scores from questions 3 to 16 and add the total to Section C of Table 12-4, at the end of this assessment.

Part III: General Risk Factors

18. Did your mother have amalgam fillings when you were conceived or when she nursed you? (*If you are under 60 years of age and do not know if your mother had amalgam fillings when you were conceived or nursed, answer **Yes**. If you are over 60 and don't know, answer **No**.*) Circle the appropriate score.

No	Yes
0	30

19. Did you receive some or most or all of your childhood vaccinations? (*If you are uncertain, it is recommended that you answer Some.*) Circle the appropriate score.

None	Some	Most	All
0	10	20	30

20. Please rate your current state of health. Circle the appropriate score.

Excellent	Good	Fair	Poor
0	10	20	30

21. On an average monthly basis, how often would you say you eat mercury-containing fish, such as Mediterranean tuna, shark, swordfish, or freshwater varieties such as trout, bass and pike? Circle the appropriate score.

Never	Less than once/month	1-5 times/month	5 or more times/month
0	5	10	15

22. Questions 17 to 20 are your *General Risk Factor* scores. Please total the scores from questions 17 to 20 and <u>add the total</u> to Section D in Table 12-4, at the end of this assessment.

PART IV: Mercury-related Symptoms

Consult Table 12-1 on Mercury-related symptoms. If you consistently have any of these symptoms, or if you would consider the symptom to be severe, please place a score of **15** next to the symptom. If you experience the symptom only occasionally, place a score of **10** next to it. If you seldom experience the symptom, mark a **5** next to it. **In each case, the symptom should be current. Please DO NOT assess a score for a symptom you have not had within the past year.**

Table 12-1

Common Symptoms of Chronic Mercury Poisoning

Emotions
Aggressiveness
Anger
Anxiety
Confusion
Depression
Fear (Recurrent)
Hallucinations

Muscles & Joints
Cramping
Joint Pain
Muscle Pain
Weakness

Neurological & Mental
Tremors
Lack Of Concentration
Learning Disorders
Memory Loss
Numbness
Slurred Speech

Oral/Throat
Bad Breath
Burning Sensation
Chronic Cough
Gingivitis/Bleeding Gums
Leukoplakia (White Patches)
Metallic Taste
Sore Throat
Ulcers of Oral Cavity

Nose
Inflammation
Sinusitis
Stuffy Nose
Excessive Mucus Formation

Head
Dizziness
Faintness
Headaches (Recurrent)
Ringing In Ears

Digestive System
Colitis
Loss of Appetite
Weight Loss
Nausea/Vomiting

Energy Levels
Apathy
Chronic Fatigue
Restlessness

Heart
Anemia
Chest Pain
Rapid or Irregular Heartbeat

Lungs
Asthma
Bronchitis
Chest Congestion
Shortness of Breath

Other
Allergies
Anorexia
Excessive Blushing
Genital Discharge
Gland Swelling
Hair Loss
Illnesses (Recurrent)
Insomnia
Loss of Sense of Smell
Perspiration (Excessive)
Kidney Failure
Skin (Cold and Clammy)
Skin Problems
Vision Problems (Tunnel Vision)
Edema (Water Retention)

Please add your scores for a total score for Mercury-related Symptoms and place the total in Section E of Table 12-4, at the end of this assessment.

PART V: Mercury-related Diseases

Please refer to Table 12-2 on diseases related to mercury poisoning. If you currently have any of the diseases listed, even if it is in its early stages, give yourself **30** points for each disease you currently have. If you have had a disease listed, but have not experienced symptoms within the past year, give yourself **15** points for each disease you have had.

Table 12-2

Diseases Related to Mercury Poisoning

Acrodynia	Emphysema
Alzheimer's	Fibromyalgia
Amyotrophic Lateral Sclerosis	Hormonal Dysfunction
Asthma	Intestinal Dysfunction
Arthritis	Immune System Disorders
Autism	Kidney Disease
Candida	Learning Disorders
Cardiovascular Disease	Liver Disorders
Crohn's Disease	Metabolic Encephalopathy
Chronic Fatique Syndrome	Multiple Sclerosis
Depression	Reproductive Disorders
Developmental Defects	Parkinson's
Diabetes	Senile Dementia
Eczema	Thyroid Disease

Please add your scores together to provide a total score for Mercury-related Diseases and place the total in Section F in Table 12-4, at the end of this assessment.

PART VI: Other Debilitating Diseases

Next, for every serious disease you currently have that is not listed above, add **30** points. For example, if you have Hodgkin's disease or any type of cancer, give yourself an additional **30** points. If you have had a debilitating disease that is not listed in the above table, but have not experienced symptoms within the past year, give yourself **15** points

Please add your scores together to provide a total score for Other Debilitating Diseases and place the total in Section G of Table 12-4, at the end of this assessment.

PART VII: OCCUPATION AND PRODUCT RISKS

Next, please review the Table 12-3 of products that may contain mercury. If you are occupationally involved in a manufacturing process that uses mercury in any form, put **30** points in Table 12-4 at the end of this survey. If you are employed by a company that uses mercury in its products, but you don't work in production or are not directly exposed to the products, enter **15** points.

Table 12-3

Industrial Uses of Mercury

Acetaldehyde Production	Germicidal Agents
Antiseptics	Histology Products
Antisyphilitic Agents	Ink Manufacturing
Bactericides	Infrared Detectors
Barometers	Insecticidal Products
Batteries	Manometers
Bronzing	Mercury Amalgam Fillings
Calibration Devices	Metal Mining and Production
Chemical Laboratories	Mirror Silvering
Chlor-alkali Production	Mercury and Neon Lamps
Cosmetics	Paints
Diaper Products	Paper Pulp Products
Electric Switches	Pathology Reagents
Electroplating	Perfumes
Embalming Agents	Photography Reagents
Explosives	Polyurethane Foam Production
Fabric Softeners	Seed Preservation
Farming Industry	Semi-Conductor Cells
Finger Printing Products	Spermicidal Jellies
Floor Wax and Polish	Tattooing Inks
Fluorescent Lamps	Taxidermy
Fossil Fuel Production/Combustion	Thermometers
Fungicidal Products	Vaccine Preservatives
Fur Hat Processing	Wood Preservatives

Please add your scores together to provide a total score for Occupation and Product Risks and place the total in Section H of Table 12-4, at the end of this assessment.

PART VIII: ENVIRONMENTAL EXPOSURE

Finally, add **30** points if you qualify for any of the following:

- you live downwind from a fossil-fuel burning plant, such as a power-generating facility;

- you live in an area proximal to any other facility that releases mercury in any form into the atmosphere, such as a refinery, pulp mill or mining/smelting operation;

- you live in an area where heavy metals are released into an aquatic environment from industrial activities and where the water is also used for recreational, domestic, or irrigation purposes; or

- you live near croplands or agricultural lands where pesticides and herbicides are employed.

Please add your scores together to provide a <u>total score</u> for Environmental Exposure and place the <u>total</u> in Section I of Table 12-4, at the end of this assessment.

Calculations

To complete the assessment, go to Table 12-4 and work through the calculations. First, calculate your **Total Amalgam Risk** by multiplying Sections A, B and C and placing the answer in the space provided. Next, add up all your risk factors from Sections D to I to calculate your **Total General Risk**.

Finally, in Table 12-4, add your **Total Amalgam Risk** and your **Total General Risk** to arrive at a final figure. This is your *TOTAL RISK*. Using this score, consult with Table 12-5 to determine your mercury Risk Category.

Table 12-4

Adding the Points

Section	Score Categories	Score Values
A	Amalgam Filling Score (place a "0" for no amalgams)	
B	Time Factor Score (place a "0" for no amalgams)	
C	Personal Risk Factors Score (Q 3-16)	

Total Amalgam Risk:

Take your scores from each of the above categories and
multiply them to obtain your Total Amalgam Risk score.

A (___) x B (___) x C (___) = _____

For non-amalgam respondents this total will equal Zero

D	General Risk Factors Score (Q 17-20)	
E	Mercury-related Symptoms	
F	Mercury-related Diseases	
G	Other Debilitating Diseases	
H	Occupational and Product Risks	
I	Environmental Exposure	

Total General Risk:

Now, add the scores from Sections D to I to obtain your overall General Risk score.

D (___) + E (___) + F (___) + G (___) + H (___) + I (___) = ____

Total Risk

Finally, add your Total Amalgam Risk to your Total General Risk,
calculated above, to obtain your Total Combined Risk:

Total Amalgam Risk (___) + Total General Risk (___) = TOTAL RISK (___)

Finally, using the above score, consult with Table 12-5 to determine your Mercury Risk Category

Determine Your Risk Category

The final step is to determine your risk category by comparing your total risk score to table 12-5.

Table 12-5

Risk Categories

Category	Points
Low	0-150
Medium	151-300
High	301+

Final Analysis

This mercury risk assessment will provide you with a general indication of your level of risk of mercury exposure. It is a valuable exercise in understanding the various means through which mercury can compromise your health. It is also useful in identifying habits, such as regularly drinking hot liquids and chewing gum, which you should avoid until all of your fillings have been safely removed.

Please, remember that the risk categories outlined in the preceding assessment are subjective, relative, and not scientifically exact. Nevertheless, if you find yourself in the medium- or high-risk category, it is cause for concern. A high score should encourage you to be tested for mercury, have your fillings removed, and participate in a mercury detoxification program.

CHAPTER 13

What's Next For You?

"When you come to a fork in the road—take it!"
— Yogi Berra,
New York Yankees

You now have the knowledge you need to make an informed choice about amalgam fillings. Will you have them removed and begin enjoying the benefits of improved health, or will you keep them in place and hope for the best?

If you are not convinced that amalgam fillings are a health hazard, you can take comfort in knowing that you objectively considered all the information. On the other hand, if you have decided to have your amalgams replaced with a nontoxic composite, you should learn the safest way to do so. You may also want to participate in a mercury detoxification program.

MERCURY-FREE DENTISTRY

Your first step is to find a qualified mercury-free dentist. Currently, less than ten percent of practicing general dentists in the United States promote themselves as mercury-free. Although that number is increasing yearly, finding a mercury-free dentist is not as easy as it should be.

Mercury-free dentists may use other names to describe themselves, such as holistic, biological, alternative, or metal-free dentists. The distinctions are not always clear and there are no standards specifically governing mercury-free dentists. Generally speaking, dentists who identify themselves as biological or holistic are concerned with more than just the mechanics of dentistry. They have a keen awareness of the relationship of oral health to the general health of the body and seek to provide alternatives to standard dental treatment that employ a more holistic (whole body) approach. Alternative-care dentists are likely to indicate that they are mercury-free, but may also provide many of the other services that biological dentists offer. Those promoting themselves as metal-free will certainly be mercury-free, but you will have to ask what other services they offer.

The following is a list of therapies that these dentists may offer in addition to mercury-free dental treatment. Depending on your needs and the dentist's evaluation, you may be provided with the option of one or more of these adjunct therapies to support your overall treatment. On request, any dentist offering these therapies will be happy to explain them to you.

Table 13-1

Services Offered by Mercury-Free Dentists

Acupuncture	Heavy Metal Detoxification
Applied Kinesiology	Homeopathy
Biocompatibility Testing	Myofunctional Therapy
Cavitation Surgery	Neural Therapy
Cranial Sacral Cavitations	Nonmetal Restorations
Electrodermal Testing	Nutritional Therapies

One of the greatest benefits a mercury-free dentist can offer is the safe removal of amalgam fillings. Before having your fillings removed, verify that your dentist uses the accepted IAOMT (International Academy of Oral Medicine and Toxicology) protocol.

To make your search for a dentist as easy as possible, I have enlisted the help of Dr. Tom McGuire to compile a worldwide database of mercury-free dental services. You can obtain free access to this valuable information on our Web site, *www.mercuryfreenow.com*. The site also includes a description of the accepted protocol for removing amalgam fillings.

COST OF REPLACEMENT

For many seeking amalgam removal, the cost of the procedure is of primary concern. It is one thing to understand that these fillings are harmful and another to have to deal with the financial challenge of the replacement procedure. For some people, unless they are on a dental insurance program that will pay for removal and replacement, the cost of this procedure can be a deciding factor. For those concerned about cost, keep in mind that amalgam fillings are not permanent and will have to be replaced at some point. The average lifespan of an amalgam filling is about eight years, and often they do not last that long. In any case, you will eventually have to have your amalgam fillings replaced.

The composite fillings that are most commonly used to replace amalgam fillings are anywhere from 20 to 100 percent more expensive; however, the cost of removing these fillings will never be less than it is today. The longer you wait to have your amalgams replaced, the more it will cost you. Moreover, the longer amalgam fillings are in your teeth, the more your health will be compromised by the accumulating mercury. Do not wait until your amalgam fillings break down to have them replaced—do it now.

If amalgam removal sounds expensive, consider the cost of medical treatment for chronic degenerative disease. The future costs of treating mercury-related symptoms and diseases far outweigh the immediate costs of having your fillings replaced. For those who remain in the low-risk category, this consideration may not be significant; for others, future mercury-related medical costs will be substantial, far outdistancing the cost of removal and replacement.

> *If your health deteriorates because of the mercury leaking from your fillings, not only will you spend significantly more money on medical care, but your ability to love and enjoy life to the fullest could be diminished substantially.*

Another consideration is your quality of life-something you cannot put a price on. If your health deteriorates because of the mercury leaking from your fillings, not only will you spend significantly more money on medical care, but your ability to love and enjoy life to the fullest could be diminished substantially.

You are now aware of the many factors that determine the extent of the acute and chronic health effects of mercury poisoning. Also, remember that mercury poisoning is the *Great Masquerader*—it is impossible to predict the way in which it will affect you. For that reason, if you are in the high end of the low-risk category or above, you should have your amalgam fillings removed as soon as possible.

In particular, if you are a woman contemplating bearing children, you should make every effort to have all of your amalgams removed at least one month or longer before trying to conceive. In addition, you should participate in a mercury detoxification program—by taking these preventive measures, not only will you improve your health, you will help ensure that your child has the best chance possible for a normal and healthy life.

> *If you are a woman contemplating bearing children, you should absolutely have your amalgams removed at least six months before trying to conceive.*

PREVENTION AND INTERVENTION

Prevention is the key to health. In a perfect world, taking preventive action means eliminating the possibility of something harmful happening to you. In the real world, that is not always possible; consequently, we should also practice *intervention*. Once you learn that something is harmful, you should immediately intervene to stop it from doing further damage.

Like a mother whose quick actions rescue her children from danger, we must intervene when we find we have placed our own bodies in harm's way. In the case of mercury poisoning, this practical philosophy of intervention means removing the toxin and providing your body with the nutrients required to restore itself to optimal health.

For those already expressing symptoms or diseases related to mercury poisoning, the sooner you practice intervention the easier it will be for your body to remove whatever mercury has accumulated and to reverse, as much as possible, the damage done. However, even if you have not yet experienced symptoms and diseases, why wait until you actually exhibit signs of mercury poisoning before you act? Why not think smart and act now—practice prevention!

Protect Your Children

If you are a parent or a parent-to-be, I urge you to take this same proactive approach with your children. If your child has tooth decay and must have fillings, tell your dentist that you will not allow the use of mercury amalgam, regardless of whether your child's teeth are baby teeth or permanent. If there is any attempt on your dentist's part to convince you otherwise—and be prepared for this, as there likely will be—let your dentist know that you are unwilling to accept an argument in favor of amalgam fillings. If this does not resolve the issue, then take your business elsewhere and find a mercury-free dentist who respects your child's health and your wishes. Unfortunately, some dentists forget that they are in *your* service—not the other way around.

With the exception of baby teeth, which will soon be replaced by permanent ones, if your child already has amalgam fillings, please make every effort to have them safely replaced as early as possible. Also, have your child evaluated to determine if he or she has any symptoms that could be related to mercury poisoning. This is particularly important with learning disorders or any signs of depletion of the immune system, such as allergic reactions and low resistance to infections. If uncertain, ask your physician to conduct a fecal-metals test for your child.

Reduce Exposure Prior to Removal

Reducing exposure to mercury before your fillings are removed is very beneficial. This is particularly important for pregnant and nursing mothers; they should *never* have amalgam fillings removed during pregnancy or while nursing. By practicing the following methods, you will decrease the amount of mercury that enters your body, and your body will be more effective at removing the mercury that has already accumulated.

Consumption of Foods

There are a number of ways to reduce stimulation of your amalgam fillings when you eat. First, make a conscientious effort to limit your daily food intake to your main meals until your fillings have been removed. I strongly encourage you to eliminate snacking; but, if you do snack, limit your consumption of abrasive and acidic foods and drinks until your fillings have been removed. Use a straw and rinse well after eating. Better yet, take a high-quality chewable calcium supplement, such as offered by USANA Health Sciences, to neutralize the acids in the mouth.

Also, limit your daily intake of hot items or let them cool before consuming. Rinsing your teeth with cool water immediately after consuming hot foods or liquids is also advisable. Seeds and nuts are generally regarded as healthful foods; however, avoid them, if possible, until your fillings have been removed or use a food processor to grind the nuts and seeds. Nut butters, such as almond butter or pumpkin-seed butter, will also minimize amalgam abrasion compared to the whole nut or seed.

Baths and Saunas

Any activity that increases your body temperature will also elevate the temperature of your amalgams and consequently increase the release of mercury vapor. Before your fillings are removed, whenever you take a hot bath or sauna, rinse your teeth with cool (not cold) water throughout the process. After rinsing, spit out the water to avoid swallowing any mercury that was taken up by the saliva. This will prevent it from being transformed into the more toxic organic forms.

Brushing

Toothpaste captures some of the mercury vapor that amalgam fillings release when they are brushed. Until your fillings have been removed, always use toothpaste when you brush your teeth. Avoid brushing the surfaces of amalgam fillings; however, brushing at the junction of the filling and the tooth, where decay often occurs, is acceptable. Do not use an electric toothbrush on amalgam surfaces until your fillings have been removed and replaced with biologically friendly composites.

Bruxism

If you are a tooth grinder, I strongly suggest that you consider using a soft night guard to prevent tooth-to-amalgam and amalgam-to-amalgam grinding. If the delay in removing your fillings will be longer than a year, consider the use of a more durable night guard. This will significantly reduce the amount of mercury vapor that you could be exposed to during that time.

Chewing Gum

The message here is short and simple: DO NOT chew gum until all your amalgam fillings have been removed. The avoidance of gum chewing has the added advantage of reducing the unnecessary intake of refined sugars that stimulate further tooth decay.

Cleaning and Polishing

Instruct your dental hygienist and dentist that you do not want to use the *Cavitron*® or any other ultrasonic tooth cleaner on the surfaces of your amalgam fillings. This does not mean that you should not have your teeth cleaned. Hand-held cleaning instruments, which can be used selectively, minimize the amount of heat generated in the cleaning process. It is also important not to have the surfaces of your amalgam fillings polished after cleaning, although your teeth can still be polished as long as the amalgam fillings are avoided.

> *Following these simple recommendations will reduce your exposure to mercury vapor and amalgam particles.*

Smoking

Smoking increases the temperature of the oral cavity and enhances the leakage of mercury from amalgams. It also adds cadmium, another heavy metal that magnifies mercury's toxicity. So, if you are a smoker—STOP. You have heard a million reasons why you should quit smoking. Now you have heard a million and one.

Stress

While it is not always easy, make every effort to reduce your stress level during the processes of filling removal and detoxification. Stress only adds to your oxidative load and furthers the damaging effects of mercury. There are many good publications available which address the issue of stress management and provide a variety of natural and healthful means of managing this unwanted complication. Do your best to stay positive and visualize, daily, a healthy future without the toxic burden of your amalgam fillings.

Following these simple recommendations will reduce your exposure to mercury vapor and amalgam particles. Please do *not* be lulled into feeling that these measures will eliminate the need to have your amalgams removed. This, indeed, would be a very costly mistake.

CHAPTER 14

Health Benefits
of Removing Mercury
from the Body

"Mercury poisoning is the greatest masquerader of our time. Dentists are not in a position to see the cause-and-effect relationship of the insertion of mercury and the development of illness three to ten years later. Even the patient himself does not connect the illness to the original dental process."

— Dr. Alfred Zamm,
Environmental Medicine

The decision to remove your amalgam fillings requires both a financial and psychological commitment from you; for that reason, it should only be made with a full understanding of what health improvements can be expected, should you choose to proceed. You now understand the risks that await you, should you choose not to do so. To assist you in your decision, let us look at some of the evidence, gleaned from an extensive array of clinical studies on amalgam removal, which clearly show the health benefits that are enjoyed from removal of this poison.

CASE STUDIES

In a compilation of studies involving a total of 1,569 patients, researcher Sam Ziff has documented the improvement of disease symptoms that follows amalgam removal. Table 14-1 shows a summary of these studies. The information is based on the percentage of patients who demonstrated significant reduction or complete eradication of disease symptoms following amalgam removal. According to the data, the symptoms that show the most improvement are: a lack of energy, metallic taste, gum problems, anxiety, irritability, allergy, and depression. While before-and-after

Table 14-1

Symptom Improvement After Amalgam Removal

Percent with Symptoms	Type of Symptom	Total	Numbers Improved/Cured	Percent Improved/Cured
6	Lack Of Energy	91	88	97
17	Metallic Taste	260	247	95
8	Gum Problems	129	121	94
5	Anxiety	86	80	93
22	Depression	347	315	91
8	Irritability	132	119	90
14	Allergy	221	196	89
5	Bad Temper	81	68	89
22	Dizziness	343	301	88
6	Bloating	88	70	88
5	Chest Pains	79	69	87
34	Headaches	531	460	87
10	Irregular Heart Beat	159	139	87
45	Fatigue	705	603	86
12	Ulcers (Oral Cavity)	189	162	86
10	Nervousness	158	131	83
8	Muscle Tremor	126	104	83
15	Intestinal Problems	231	192	83
8	Numbness	118	97	82
17	Lack Of Concentration	270	216	80
12	Insomnia	187	146	78
7	Multiple Sclerosis	113	86	76
17	Memory Loss	265	193	73
29	Vision Problems	462	289	63
6	High Or Low Blood Pressure	99	53	54

studies such as these cannot control for all variables (including the placebo effect, where a patient improves because (s)he simply *believes* it will happen), the sole defining experimental variable was amalgam removal. In addition, the overwhelmingly positive responses provide strong subjective evidence of substantial improvement following removal.

An excellent study by Swiss dentist Paul Engel[1] demonstrated significant improvements of symptoms related to mercury toxicity following amalgam removal. The test subjects were patients who had previously received amalgam fillings, placed by Engel before he became aware of the health hazards of mercury. The purpose of the study was to determine what symptoms existed before amalgam removal and which of those improved after removal. As the patients did not undergo postoperative detoxification, it is believed that the improvements reported were solely the result of amalgam filling removal.

Engel evaluated 53 symptoms in 75 patients. Each patient had one or more symptoms, which ranged from one case of diabetes to 68 complaints of chronic headaches and migraines. Other symptoms included gastrointestinal problems, neck tension, dizziness, allergies, vision disturbances, chronic back pain, psychological disorders, and joint pain. Eighty percent of the patients reported significant to strong improvement (indicated by the mitigation or complete elimination of symptoms) after removal of the amalgam fillings. About nine percent reported marginal improvement, seven percent reported no improvement and less than two percent reported a worsening of symptoms.

In a recent survey of 60 patients who underwent amalgam removal for a variety of health-related reasons, the findings reveal that 78 percent of respondents were "satisfied" or "very satisfied" with the results, while less than ten percent were disappointed. Headaches and backaches appeared to respond best to amalgam removal; fatigue, memory loss and concentration problems also showed demonstrable improvement. Other health challenges that improved significantly included joint and muscle pain; stomach, bowel and bladder complaints; depression; food and chemical sensitivities; numbness of limbs; and vision problems.[2]

At Sweden's Karolinska Institute, a 1998 study evaluated 12 patients who underwent amalgam removal. Despite a transient increase in the levels of mercury in the blood and urine within 48 hours following amalgam removal, an exponential decline in mercury levels occurred thereafter. Sixty days following removal of dental amalgams, mercury levels in the blood and urine plummeted 40 percent. In subjects who were followed for three years, the mercury levels continued to recede to the levels of subjects without any dental amalgams.[3] The study revealed that, subsequent to amalgam removal, the body continues to flush mercury from its system until body fluid levels eventually reach those of individuals who have had no previous amalgam exposure. However, no indication was given regarding residual mercury levels in the CNS or other body tissues.

> *Subsequent to amalgam removal, the body continues to flush mercury from its system until body fluid levels eventually reach those of individuals who have had no previous amalgam exposure.*

The findings of the Karolinska study are also supported by an earlier study, conducted at the Umea University, Sweden.[4] In this study, amalgam restorations were removed from 18 subjects in a single treatment session in which a rubber dam (which protects the patient from mercury vapor and amalgam fragments) was used, and from ten subjects in which a rubber dam was not used. After removal of amalgams, only the no-rubber-dam group showed significant increases in mercury levels in the blood, indicating that mercury vapor or elemental mercury had been absorbed. One year later, the mercury levels in the blood and urine had sunk significantly below the preremoval levels for both groups: blood mercury levels had declined by 52 percent and urine mercury levels had plummeted by 76 percent.

The Umea study shows that the removal of amalgam fillings has a statistically significant impact on the reduction of levels of mercury in the blood and urine. The study also confirms that the use of a rubber dam during removal of the fillings reduces the transient elevation of mercury, observed in several other studies.

OTHER STUDIES

A 1994 study by Bergerow and coworkers provides further evidence of the reduction in the body burden of mercury following removal of dental amalgams. The researchers investigated long-term mercury excretion at various time intervals following amalgam removal. They noted that, before removal, the level of urinary excretion of mercury correlated with the number of amalgam fillings. In the immediate postremoval phase and up to six days after removal, urine mercury levels jumped 30 percent. However, within 12 months following amalgam removal, the participants showed substantially lower urinary mercury levels that were comparable to those subjects who had never had dental amalgams.[5] Keep in mind that the levels of mercury in body fluids, such as blood and urine, do not correlate with the residual body burden; however, they are a reliable indicator of exposure.

In other research conducted on blood mercury levels following amalgam removal, investigators found a statistically significant drop in blood levels at 18 weeks following extraction. Although removal of the amalgams provided an additional exposure, the added mercury burden was rapidly cleared from the blood.[6]

Molin and coworkers evaluated mercury levels following replacement of mercury amalgams with gold inlays. The findings reveal that, despite a significant but transient elevation of blood and urinary mercury immediately following amalgam removal, plasma and urinary mercury levels dropped dramatically. Within twelve months, levels had receded to 50 percent and 25 percent respectively of the initial values for the experimental group.[7] Similar findings have been confirmed in several other studies.[8,9]

AMALGAM REMOVAL SUPPORTED BY MERCURY DETOXIFICATION

As the two following studies illustrate, improvements in symptoms and overall health are greater and take place sooner when filling removal and replacement is combined with a detoxification program.

In a study of symptoms of mercury toxicity, 35 people who had previously been told that their cognitive deficits and mood swings were psychosomatic underwent amalgam removal.[10] The range of health problems reported by this group included chronic fatigue syndrome, *Candida* (a recurring yeast infection), allergies, migraines, and chronic or recurring flu-symptoms indicative of a compromised immune system.

Of the 32 individuals who underwent amalgam removal, 90 percent reported lasting benefits, and of the 30 subjects who completed both amalgam removal and detoxification, 70 percent experienced a full return to health and the activities of normal daily life. Only one person who followed the amalgam removal and detoxification protocols failed to experience any lasting improvement. The three individuals who did not have their amalgams removed remained ill and felt that they were deteriorating. Eight other participants reported an initial recovery from symptoms that they attributed to mercury poisoning. This was followed by the appearance of latent symptoms that only surfaced once the most overt symptoms had been resolved. Such occurrences have been reported elsewhere and are indicative of the complex nature of mercury toxicity. Like the skin of an onion, once you peel away the outer layer (in this case the primary disease symptoms), you expose the inner layers (secondary and tertiary symptoms), each of which must then be resolved accordingly.

> *Like the skin of an onion, once you peel away the outer layer (in this case the primary disease symptoms), you expose the inner layers (secondary and tertiary symptoms).*

In another study, Lindh and coworkers[11] evaluated the responses of 776 people to the removal of their amalgam fillings. Similar to the studies by Ziff, researchers focused on the abatement of symptoms and improvements in the quality of life. The subjects suffered from an array of symptoms, including neurological, psychiatric, oral, and general health issues. More than 70 percent of those who underwent both filling removal and detoxification reported a substantial recovery and an increased quality of life.

INTERPRETING THE DATA

The subjects participating in all of the above studies had a number of symptoms and diseases associated with mercury poisoning. As the evidence clearly shows, a very high percentage showed significant improvement following removal of their mercury amalgams, even though these individuals were not medically treated for any specific disease. Quite simply, the only treatment they received was to have the source of the problem removed—the body, itself, did the healing.

Moreover, the majority of participants showed dramatic improvement; only a small percentage showed marginal improvement or no improvement at all. This is to be expected, because mercury from amalgam fillings does not cause every health issue. Also, those who did not improve were usually in the highest risk category and had the most severe, and possibly permanent, damage. As would be expected, the symptoms that improve first when amalgams are removed appear to be those that have been present for the shortest time.

All of the conditions reported in the above studies, with the exception of gum problems, would normally have been brought to the attention of a physician or other health practitioner, rather than to a dentist. Consequently, precious time and resources are frequently wasted as the physician attempts, often in vain, to isolate and identify the etiology (cause) of the problem. This can be frustrating and costly for both the patient and the healthcare system. For this reason, it behooves both physicians and dental personnel to become more acquainted with the symptoms of mercury poisoning. I strongly recommend that any patient with existing health problems who also has mercury amalgam fillings should be tested for mercury toxicity, preferably with the fecal-metals test.

> *DAMS researchers have compiled the findings of 60,000 cases of amalgam replacement, providing clear evidence of cure or significant improvement.*

EVIDENCE COMPILED BY DAMS

For over 20 years, the Dental Amalgam Mercury Syndrome group (DAMS), a U.S.-based patient support group that provides information to mercury-toxic individuals, has compiled detailed information about improvements in related diseases and illnesses following amalgam removal. In the process, DAMS has evaluated over 1,000 peer-reviewed and government studies showing that mercury is either the principal cause or a major contributing factor in over 40 chronic health conditions. DAMS research coordinators have also compiled the findings of 60,000 cases of amalgam replacement, as documented by qualified health practitioners,[12] providing clear evidence of cure or significant improvement in the following chronic conditions:

- *Autoimmune:* Alzheimer's, arthritis, chronic fatigue syndrome, Crohn's, diabetes, endometriosis, fibromyalgia, joint and muscular pain, amyotrophic lateral sclerosis (Lou Gehrig's disease), lupus, multiple sclerosis, muscle tremor, scleroderma, Parkinson's disease.

- *Cardiovascular:* angina, atherosclerosis, hypertension, tachycardia.

- *Eye:* astigmatism, cataracts, color blindness, inflammation, iritis, macular degeneration, myopia, vision disturbances.

- *Hormonal:* adrenal problems, alopecia/hair loss, chronic chills, Hashimoto's disease, hypothyroidism, urinary/prostrate problems.

- *Immune system:* allergies, antibiotic-resistant infections, asthma, susceptibility to infection, multiple chemical sensitivities, sinus problems, eczema, psoriasis and other skin conditions.

- *Neurological:* mood disorders, attention deficit disorder (ADD), anger, anxiety, mental confusion, depression, dizziness and vertigo, dyslexia, epilepsy, chronic headaches and migraines, hearing loss, insomnia, learning disabilities, memory loss, neuropathy and paresthesia (an abnormal tingling or burning sensation of the skin), schizophrenia, suicidal thoughts, tinnitus.

- *Oral:* amalgam tattoos, halitosis, metallic taste in mouth, oral keratosis (pre-cancer), oral lichen planus, periodontal diseases.

- *Reproductive:* birth defects, developmental disabilities, infertility, learning disabilities and low IQ (in children), postmenstrual syndrome, reduced sperm count, spontaneous abortions.

- *Stomach and digestive:* Crohn's, leaky gut, malabsorption of essential minerals and essential fatty acids.

The studies that the DAMS project evaluated were not based solely on subjective anecdotal information. These case studies were unique in that the patients' health professionals documented both the original condition and its improvement.

THE VALUE OF ANECDOTAL EVIDENCE

The use of anecdotal evidence, such as has been employed in several of the above studies, is not a recognized standard for scientific inquiry as it does not conclusively prove cause-and-effect. However, the findings are extremely important to anyone who has experienced genuine relief from a symptom or the eradication of a disease as a result of amalgam removal. Anyone whose chest pains and mental confusion have suddenly disappeared because their fillings are now history is not going to be interested in the nuances of scientific methodology. Their fillings were removed and their symptoms disappeared. To them, mercury toxicity was the culprit, pure and simple. What's more, they were right!

SAFE REMOVAL OF AMALGAM FILLINGS

Amalgam fillings release the greatest amounts of mercury vapor when they are placed and removed. Consequently, following a safe removal protocol is crucial, especially if you are allergic to mercury, have a depleted immune system, or exhibit symptoms of mercury poisoning. For example, if you are allergic to mercury, removing your fillings without the proper protocol could expose you to mercury vapor levels high enough to trigger a severe allergic reaction. Safe removal procedures can reduce your mercury exposure by as much as 90 percent.

If you are unable to find a dentist who is mercury-free, I strongly recommend that you insist that the standardized IAOMT protocol be followed. This will protect you from excessive mercury exposure while your fillings are being removed. To augment detoxification *before* your fillings are replaced, it is vital that you supplement with a high-quality nutritional product that has advanced amounts of vitamins, minerals and antioxidants. I recommend the *Mega Antioxidant* and *Chelated Minerals* formulations available through USANA Health Sciences. Daily supplementation with these products will help capture and remove much of the mercury that you will unavoidably absorb during the replacement procedure. I view this as an integral and vital part of a preremoval detoxification program.

> *Be careful. Conventional dentists are not likely familiar with safe removal protocols and may advise you that this is an unnecessary precaution.*

Be careful. Conventional dentists are not likely familiar with safe removal protocols and, if asked, may advise you that this is an unnecessary precaution. Most dentists may not be concerned about the amount of mercury to which you are exposed; however, many dentists are having second thoughts about the mercury amalgam issue and will want to know what the IAOMT protocol entails. They may even be willing to take the necessary steps to comply with it. However, before you consent, there are additional factors to consider.

First, find out how much experience your dentist has in placing composite fillings. Dentists who practice mercury-free dentistry will certainly be more experienced with these biologically friendly composites than will conventional dentists. Because mercury-free dentists use composite fillings extensively, they are also more likely to keep abreast of the latest in composite materials and techniques. Composite-filling development is now in its 7th generation, and manufacturers are constantly improving the technology. Consequently, to avoid paying today's prices for a composite filling made of yesterday's materials, use a dentist who is knowledgeable about the latest composite fillings and is skilled in placing them.

ADVANTAGES OF DETOXIFICATION

Once your fillings have been safely removed and replaced, your body will be able to focus on removing the accumulated mercury. How efficiently it will do this depends on your present state of health, the strength of your detoxification and immune systems, your current body burden of mercury, and where the poison is in your body. The medium- and high-risk groups will benefit by participating in a scientifically based mercury detoxification program. If you are in the medium- or high-risk category, as determined by the mercury risk assessment provided in Chapter 12, you can be certain that your body has been depleted of antioxidants. Consequently, you will have difficulty stopping mercury's damage and removing the accumulated toxin. Remember, your body cannot fully begin to heal the damage done by mercury until the poison has been removed from your teeth.

At *Sanoviv Medical Institute*, Dr. McGuire and I, along with my dedicated research staff, have developed what I believe is the most effective mercury detoxification program available today—I strongly recommend it.

The program provides complete details on how to have your amalgam fillings removed safely and how to effectively remove mercury from your body. Our approach is to start low and go slow; the program is based on our conviction that you should not have to get sick to get well. The goal is not just to get rid of the mercury, but also to insure that your body has everything essential for it to heal.

For more detailed information on the subject of detoxification, I refer you to a book I am currently writing with Dr. Tom McGuire, *Your Complete Guide to Mercury Detoxification: How to Safely Remove Mercury from Your Teeth and Body*. This guide is designed to allow you to complete the mercury removal and detoxification program on your own or with the support of a health professional. *Your Complete Guide to Mercury Detoxification* will become an essential resource for everyone who wishes to remove toxic fillings from their teeth and get rid of the accumulated mercury from their bodies.

The sooner you make the decision to remove your amalgams, the sooner your body can get on with the task of healing itself.

> *You will never know how much your health has been affected by this poison until you remove it from your body.*

CHAPTER 15

On the Firing Line

"One of these days there's going to be a mammoth lawsuit about mercury fillings similar to one that's already been filed in Canada. It's going to be bigger than what we've seen over tobacco. It's going to hit people like a Mack truck that putting mercury in their teeth amounts to putting poison in their mouths. Once they realize that in no uncertain terms, they're going to be angry."
— Dr. Charles Williamson,
Toxic Studies Institute

In a position statement, released January 8th, 2002, the ADA describes dental amalgam as a "safe, affordable and durable material that has been used to restore the teeth of over 100 million Americans."[1] In response, the International Academy of Oral Medicine and Toxicology (IAOMT) charges that the ADA has utterly failed to support its position with hard scientific data. According to the IAOMT, this failure has resulted in inadequate protection of the public and exposure of the membership of the ADA to personal harm due to amalgam usage.[2]

The ADA claims that, while mercury is toxic at high concentrations, when combined with other metals, such as silver, tin and copper, it reacts to form a biologically inactive material. The weight of scientific evidence confirms that, far from being biologically inactive, amalgam fillings constantly release mercury vapor that travels through the oral mucosa to the neural pathways and into the brain—an absorption route that effectively delivers more mercury to the brain than eating it.[3]

The ADA concedes that very small quantities of mercury vapor are absorbed by the body; they assert, however, that there is no evidence associating this absorption with toxic effects. The scientific evidence declares otherwise: data compiled by several international health agencies confirm that the average daily intake of mercury from amalgams significantly exceeds the U.S. EPA guidelines for exposure and is 10 to 50 times greater than that considered safe by the U.S. Agency for Toxic Substances and Disease Registry (ATSDR) and Health Canada.[4,5]

The ADA attempts to deflect the issue of mercury from dental amalgam by implicating the consumption of fish as a major source of mercury exposure. The association argues that you may be exposed to more mercury from fish than from amalgam. The scientific evidence, confirmed through autopsies of people with fillings and countless clinical studies, reveals that the major source of mercury, by far, is the mercury released from dental amalgams. Exposure to amalgam fillings amounts to approximately 50 to 90 percent of the total exposure, with the average exposure about 80 percent.[6] Dr. Pierre Blais, former risk analyst with Health Canada, has publicly admonished governments who express concern over picograms (extremely small amounts) of mercury in foods, but look the other way when milligrams of mercury—one *billion* times more—are implanted directly into a child's teeth.

The ADA wants dentists to reassure patients who express concern about amalgam that it is approved as a "safe and effective" dental material. In fact, there is no approval by the ADA or any other body.[7] Amalgam is a reaction product, compounded by the individual dentist, and consequently it cannot be approved or certified. In addition, the ADA claim of confidence that the U.S. Food and Drug Administration (FDA) classified amalgam as an approved dental device is false.[8] The FDA, in fact, has

> *The fact that over 100 million fillings are placed into the mouths of Americans each year is not cause for assurance; rather, it is cause for alarm.*

actively refused to classify the set-amalgam product.[9] Also in Canada, Dr. Richard Tobin, Director of the Medical Services Division, Health Canada, rebuked the Canadian Dental Association (CDA) for disseminating similar false statements which suggested that dental amalgam was approved by Health Canada.[10]

The ADA states: "We wish the public to be as certain as we are that dental amalgam is safe, and we will pursue this matter until that certainty is assured."[11] The wording of this statement confirms that the ADA has a biased agenda. The process of scientific inquiry *demands* neutrality; it does not seek a predetermined outcome. To the ADA, there can be only one resolution to the question of amalgam fillings being a health hazard—the one it has favored for almost 150 years. Perhaps this explains why the ADA has never provided any scientific support for its position. I have exhaustively surveyed the arena and have been unable to find a single scientific report by the ADA, the FDA or any other agency confirming the safety of mercury amalgam. Such an absence is revealing in itself.

> *Responsible science requires us to ask: "What other profession would take pride in the fact that it continues to use the same primitive practices first employed over 200 years ago, particularly when they are inhumane?*

The ADA contends that amalgam has been used for over 150 years and has established a solid track record for safety and efficacy. The fact that over 100 million fillings are placed into the mouths of Americans each year is not cause for assurance; rather, it is cause for alarm. Responsible science requires us to ask, "What other profession would take pride in the fact that it continues to use the same primitive practices first employed over 200 years ago, particularly when they are inhumane? Indeed, what has hindered the ADA's progress in their own research and development of modern, safe alternatives to mercury amalgams?"

The fact is, 100 years ago few people had amalgam fillings and, with an average lifespan of only 50 years, those who had them likely did not live long enough to suffer the chronic effects of neurotoxicity. It is the current generation of aging baby boomers, born at the time amalgam use went mainstream and who have lived most of their lives with mercury fillings, which has become the great amalgam experiment. Let there be no doubt: there will be absolute hell to pay when the Boomers come to realize that they are running the risk of Alzheimer's disease—and largely because the dental industry was too busy lining its pockets to worry about the health of a nation.

> *Let there be no doubt: there will be absolute hell to pay when the Boomers come to realize that they are running the risk of Alzheimer's disease.*

The ADA knows that an admission of error is, by implication, an admission of guilt, and to admit guilt is to expose the association and its membership to liability. Better to obfuscate and delay, rather than own up to the fact. Better to stall and dodge, and hope that the development of new materials will, somehow, make the amalgam issue dry up and blow away.

Perhaps this is why the ADA discourages its members from discussing the hazards of mercury with patients. It may also explain why the association has its head in the sand (or other places) when it comes to ignoring the overwhelming scientific evidence of amalgam toxicity. It also clarifies why the Association threatens its member dentists with disbarment, jeopardizing their careers and their financial futures, simply for replacing a patient's amalgams for health-related reasons.

To admit that mercury from amalgam fillings is making people sick is to accept moral and legal responsibility for generations of willful ignorance.

The ADA has a lot of explaining to do.

My Message to Dentists

"The ADA owes no legal duty of care to protect the public from allegedly dangerous products used by dentists... Dissemination of information relating to the practice of dentistry does not create a duty of care to protect the public from potential injury."
— Statement of submission by the American Dental Association, Superior Court, State of California, in and for the County of Santa Clara

This statement of submission, filed by the ADA in the Superior Court of the State of California, says it all—the ADA has already abandoned its membership.

In seeking legal protection from pending mercury-amalgam lawsuits, the ADA is attempting to mitigate the collateral damage by distancing itself from the dental community. This action leaves individual practitioners at great personal risk.

While continuing to assure you that amalgam is safe, the ADA has failed to carry the burden of proof; while encouraging you to endorse its position, the ADA penalizes you for speaking out against the known hazards of mercury; and while encouraging you to carry their message, the ADA prepares to abandon you when the chips are down.

These legal maneuvers effectively put the individual practitioner in an odious "Catch 22." If you speak out, you may be condemned by your peers through the ADA and may lose your license to practice. On the other hand, if you say nothing and continue to place amalgam fillings, you risk the possible wrath of a public litigation process that will show little mercy for blind compliance. And the ADA has made it clear that they won't be there to help—for this reason, should you continue to place amalgam fillings, you *must* make every effort to inform your patients of the dangers and obtain their signed consent.

I have absolutely no doubt that mercury amalgam will eventually be banned in the United States and Canada, as it has been in many other parts of the world. It is not a matter of *if*, but *when* this ban takes place. Although the legal implications for practicing dentists are not yet clear, it is not difficult to see that the personal liabilities could devastate your practice, your professional life, and your private life. Consider the evidence, ask the right questions, and take the right action—for yourself and your patients. Let my opinion be clear: the dental industry and the ADA have hung the dental profession out to dry.

You may want to trust the ADA, but are you willing to bet your practice and financial future? Once you take the time to examine the evidence, you will see that the ADA's position has no merit, scientifically, legally or morally. You may also come to realize that you will never be able to use the ADA's arguments as a legal defense. If you are sued and the defendant's attorney presents the court with the massive weight of evidence that indicts amalgam fillings, are you going to plead that you were just doing what the ADA told you? I'd certainly hate to hang my hat on *that* defense.

If you do nothing, then perhaps you deserve the consequences that your actions may bring. If you think that you can continue to place a known poison into your patients' mouths, I implore you to think again. Ignorance is no excuse.

For those who now harbor doubts about the safety of the amalgam fillings but are afraid to speak up, I am concerned for you. Let me assure you that you will be in far greater danger by remaining silent than by speaking up. The courts will take a dim view of any dentist who knowingly continues to expose patients to the poisonous effects of mercury when there are now safe and cost-effective alternatives. Remember, the ADA maintains that it has no legal duty of care to protect the public—or you. Consequently, should you continue to buy into the ADA's untenable position, *you* will be the one left holding the bag.

When the fix is in, it is always the little guy that takes it on the chin.

> *The courts will take a dim view of any dentist who knowingly continues to expose patients to the poisonous effects of mercury when there are now safe and cost-effective alternatives.*

My Message to You

As a dental patient and concerned citizen, there is a lot that you can do to convince the ADA and conventional dentists to change their ways and stop placing poison in people's mouths. At a personal level, you have the power to ban mercury from your mouth and to remove it from your body. Collectively, you certainly have the power to convince your state, provincial, and federal governments to ban the further use of these poisonous fillings.

After what you have learned about mercury amalgams, it would not surprise me if you are outraged at what has been allowed to happen for all these years. I fervently hope that this outrage convinces you—as it did me—to take affirmative action. I also hope that you will channel this action into protecting not only yourself but also your family and friends.

I'm asking you to help me spread the word. The following are some ideas about how you can do this.

Communicate with your dentist and let him or her know how you feel about mercury in your mouth. Ask your dentist to read this book, and if (s)he dismisses the evidence, let him or her know that *you* know what needs to be done. Then, go out and find a mercury-free dentist who understands the issue and genuinely cares about your health and well-being.

1. Make it clear to everyone you know that it is imperative to have amalgam fillings safely removed and the body detoxified of mercury.

2. If you are a U.S citizen, let your congressperson and senators know how you feel; if you are a Canadian citizen, bend the ear of your Member of Parliament or request that they help you draft a public petition to be tabled in the House of Commons that demands a ban on the use of mercury amalgam.

3. Go to our Web site at *www.mercuryfreenow.com* to be completely updated on what is happening in the world of holistic, mercury-free dentistry. You will find a list of alternative dentists, informative books, health products, tests for mercury, allergy and biocompatibility, and laboratories that perform these tests.

4. Learn all you can about *Sanoviv Medical Institute*, beginning with a visit to *www.sanoviv.com*. *Sanoviv Medical Institute* is a fully accredited, leading-edge medical facility less than one hour from San Diego. This beautiful, toxic-free facility is a rare oasis in an increasingly toxic world. Unique to Sanoviv, the *Oral Health Program* evaluates every potential dental health issue, from cavitations to toxic metals, and offers the most advanced amalgam removal and detoxification program available today.

I hope that I have provided you with the foundation from which you can arrive at your own conclusions about how amalgam fillings affect your health and the health of your family and loved ones. Remember, knowledge means choice and freedom.

On a Personal Note

When I learned that my amalgam fillings were poisoning me and that the dental industry had completely misled me, I was very upset and angry. I could not imagine how anyone could knowingly expose me to this poisonous substance. As a health professional, I sadly reached the opinion that the ADA had not only concealed this health-destroying and life-threatening issue from me, but also actively impeded dentists from giving me the information I needed to make an informed choice. To me, this defies science, logic, and common decency. One might expect this type of obfuscation from an unethical company wishing to increase profits, such as the tobacco companies, but not from an organization whose own mission statement includes a commitment "to the public's oral health, ethics, science and professional advancement." It belies any sense of concern for humankind.

I felt victimized when I realized my trust had been seriously abused. What upset me most, however, was that in my reliance on the integrity of this organization I failed to protect my children. My first thought was that I had let them down. Of course, I know that it was not my fault; I was never provided with the information that I needed to make an informed choice. My dentist made these decisions for me, and his choices were certainly not in my best interest. Realizing that anger would not resolve anything, my best recourse was to right (and write about) this wrong for myself and others. After considerable thought, I decided that there were a number of positive steps I would take.

First, I had my amalgam fillings removed and replaced with a biocompatible alternative. I followed this with a mercury detoxification program, using nutritional supplements to support my body in removing the mercury that had accumulated. I encouraged my children to do the same.

Then, I dedicated my efforts to writing this book so that others would have a chance to learn about these issues and be able to do something for themselves and their children.

I now believe I have accomplished these goals. It is my fervent wish that this book has been beneficial to you and has provided answers to questions that you may have had for a long time.

In a sense, this last chapter marks both an ending and a beginning. It is the close of my journey in presenting the evidence you need to make an informed choice about the dangers of mercury and in summoning you to get involved—for the sake of your own health as well as those you love. It is also the dawn of your journey to better health by making the decision to remove mercury from your body, and by mentoring others to do the same.

I wish you well in your efforts.

> *Love life and may you live it to the fullest, in happiness and health.*

—Dr. Myron Wentz

REFERENCES

INTRODUCTION

1 U.S. Environmental Protection Agency (EPA), 1999, "Integrated Risk Information System, National Center for Environmental Assessment, Cincinnati, Ohio, http://www.epa.gov/ncea/iris.htm.

2 Goyer RA. Toxic effects of metals, in: Caserett and Doull's Toxicology - The Basic Science of Poisons, McGraw-Hill Inc., NY, 1993.

3 Hanson M. Why is mercury toxic? Basic chemical and biochemical properties of mercury/amalgam in relation to biological effects. Proceedings of the ICBM conference, Colorado Springs, Co, 1988.

4 Chang LW, et al. Blood-brain barrier dysfunction in experimental mercury intoxication. *Acta Neuropathol* (Berl) 1972; 21(3):179-184.

5 Arvidson K. Corrosion studies of a dental gold alloy in contact with amalgam under different conditions. *Sven Tandlak Tidskr* 1975; 68(4):135-139.

6 Monnet-Tschudi F, et al. Comparison of the developmental effects of two mercury compounds on glial cells and neurons in aggregate cultures of rat telencephalon. *Brain Res* 1996; 741(1-2):52-59.

7 Huggins HA, et al. Cerebrospinal fluid protein changes in multiple sclerosis after dental amalgam removal. *Altern Med Rev*. 1998 Aug;3(4):295-300.

8 Lorscheider FL, et al. Mercury exposure from "silver" tooth fillings: emerging evidence questions a traditional dental paradigm. *FASEB J*. 1995 Apr; 9(7):504-8.

9 Hussain S, et al. Mercuric chloride-induced reactive oxygen species and its effect on antioxidant enzymes in different regions of rat brain. *J Environ Sci Health B* 1997; 32(3):395-409.

10 Bulat P, et al. Activity of glutathione peroxidase and superoxide dismutase in workers occupationally exposed to mercury. *Int Arch Occup Environ Health*. 1998 Sep; 71 Suppl:S37-9.

11 Albers JW, et al. Neurological abnormalities associated with remote occupational elemental mercury exposure. *Ann Neurol* 1988; 24(5):651-659.

12 Soleo L, et al. Effects of low exposure to inorganic mercury on psychological performance. *Br J Ind Med* 1990; 47(2):105-109.

13 Gerhard I, et al. Impact of heavy metals on hormonal and immunological factors in women with

repeated miscarriages. *Hum Reprod Update* 1998; 4(3):301-309.

14 Veltman JC, et al. Alterations of heme, cytochrome P-450, and steroid metabolism by mercury in rat adrenal. *Arch Biochem Biophys* 1986;248(2):467-478.

15 Kawada J, et al. Effects of organic and inorganic mercurials on thyroidal functions. *J Pharmacobiodyn* 1980;3(3):149-159.

16 Nylander M, et al. Mercury concentrations in the human brain and kidneys in relation to exposure from dental amalgam fillings. *Swed Dent J* 1987;11(5):179-187.

17 Lee IP, et al. Effects of mercury on spermatogenesis studied by velocity sedimentation cell separation and serial mating. *J Pharmacol Exp Ther* 1975;194(1):171-181.

18 Ogura H, et al. A comparison of the 8-hydroxydeoxyguanosine, chromosome aberrations and micronucleus techniques.... *Mutat Res* 1996;340(2-3):175-182.

19 Ronnback L,et al. Chronic encephalopathies induced by mercury or lead: aspects of underlying cellular and molecular mechanisms. *Br J Ind Med* 1992;49(4):233-240.

20 Marlowe M, et al. Main and interaction effects of metallic toxins on classroom behavior. *J Abnorm Child Psychol* 1985;13(2):185-198.

21 Moon C, et al. Main and interaction effects of metallic pollutants on cognitive functioning. *J Learn Disabil* 1985;18(4):217-221.

22 Salonen JT, et al. Intake of mercury from fish, lipid peroxidation, and the risk of myocardial infarction and coronary, cardiovascular, and any death in eastern Finnish men. *Circulation* 1995; 91(3):645-655.

23 Salonen JT, et al. Mercury accumulation and accelerated progression of carotid atherosclerosis.... *Atherosclerosis* 2000;148(2):265-273.

24 Hultman P, et al. Adverse immunological effects and autoimmunity induced by dental amalgam and alloy in mice. *FASEB J* 1994 November;8(14):1183-90.

25 Abraham JE, et al. The effect of dental amalgam restorations on blood mercury levels. *J Dent Res* 1984;63(1):71-73.

26 Snapp KR et al. The contribution of dental amalgam to mercury in blood. *J Dent Res* 1989 May;68(5):780-5

27 Zamm AV. Removal of dental mercury: often an effective treatment for very sensitive patients. *J Orthomolecular Med.* 1990;5(53):138-142.

28 Windham B. Mercury Exposure Levels from Amalgam Dental Fillings.... As cited in: http://www.vaccinationnews.com/DailyNews/August2002/MercuryExposureLevels25.htm. Accessed Jun 19, 2004.

29 Moore C. A Review of Mercury in the Environment: Its Occurrence in Marine Fish. Office of Environmental management, Marine Resources Division, South Carolina Department of Natural Resources. Nov 2000. URL: http://water.dnr.state.sc.us/marine/img/mm_paper.pdf. Accessed April 15, 2004.

CHAPTER 1

1 International Academy of Oral Medicine and Toxicology (IAOMT). A Scientific Response to the American Dental Association's Special Report.... URL: http://www.iaomt.org//documents/A%20Scientific%20Response.pdf. Accessed Aug 3, 2004.

2 Ibid.

3 Ibid.

4 Sharma RP, et al. Metals and neurotoxic effects: cytotoxicity of selected metallic compounds on chick ganglia cultures. *J Comp Pathol.* 1981;91(2):235-244.

5 Leirskar J. On the mechanism of cytotoxicity of silver and copper amalgams in a cell culture system. *Scand J Dent Res.* 1974;82(1):74-81.

6 Wedeen RP. Lead, mercury and cadmium nephropathy. *Neurotoxicology.* 1983;4(3):134-146.

7 Stock A. Die Gefährlichkeit des Quecksilberdampfes. *Z Anges Chem.* 1926;39:461-488.

8 International Academy of Oral Medicine and Toxicology (IAOMT). A Scientific Response to the American Dental Association's Special Report.... URL: http://www.iaomt.org//documents/A%20Scientific%20Response.pdf. Accessed Aug 3, 2004.

9 Stock A. Chronic mercury and amalgam intoxication. *Zahnärztl Rundsch.* 1939;10:371-377.

10 Frykholm KO. Mercury from dental amalgam. Its toxic and allergic effects and some comments on occupational hygiene. *Acta Odont Scand.* 1957;22:1-108.

11 Gay DD, et al. Chewing releases mercury from fillings. *Lancet.* 1979;1(8123):985-986.

12 Svare CW, et al. The effect of dental amalgams on mercury levels in expired air. *J Dent Res.* 1981;60(9):1668-1671.

13 Abraham JE, et al. The effect of dental amalgam restorations on blood mercury levels. *J Dent Res.* 1984;63(1):71-73.

14 Patterson JE, et al. Mercury in human breath from dental amalgams. *Bull Environ Contam Toxicol.* 1985;34(4):459-468.

15 Vimy MJ, et al. Estimation of mercury body burden from dental amalgam: computer simulation of a metabolic compartmental model. *J Dent Res.* 1986;65(12):1415-1419.

16 Langworth S, et al. Mercury exposure from dental fillings. I. Mercury concentrations in blood and urine. *Swed Dent J.* 1988;12(1-2):69-70.

17 Aronsson AM, et al. Dental amalgam and mercury. *Biol Met.* 1989;2(1):25-30.

18 Workshop: biocompatibility of metals in dentistry. National Institute of Dental Research. *J Am Dent Assoc.* 1984;109(3):469-471.

19 ANON. When your patients ask about mercury in amalgam. *J Am Dent Assoc.* 1990;120(4):395-398.

20 International Academy of Oral Medicine and Toxicology (IAOMT). A Scientific Response to the American Dental Association's Special Report.... URL: http://www.iaomt.org//documents/A%20Scientific%20Response.pdf. Accessed Aug 3, 2004.

21 Ibid.

22 O'Brian J. Mercury Amalgam Toxicity: Your next visit to the dentist may not be as innocent as you think. *Life Extension Magazine.* May 2001.

23 Y.Omura et al. Heart Disease Research Foundation, NY,NY, "Role of mercury in resistant infections and recovery after Hg detox with cilantro", Acupuncture & Electro-Theraputics Research, 20(3):195-229, 1995.

24 O'Brian J. Mercury Amalgam Toxicity: Your next visit to the dentist may not be as innocent as you think. *Life Extension Magazine.* May 2001.

25 Vimy MJ, et al. Maternal-fetal distribution of mercury (203Hg) released from dental amalgam fillings. *Am J Physiol.* 1990;258(4 Pt 2):R939-R945.

26 Willershausen-Zonnchen B, et al. [Mercury concentration in the mouth mucosa of patients with amalgam fillings]. *Dtsch Med Wochenschr.* 1992;117(46):1743-1747.

27 Gebel T, et al. Assessment of a possible genotoxic environmental risk in sheep bred on grounds with strongly elevated contents of mercury, arsenic and antimony. *Mutat Res.* 1996;368(3-4):267-274.

28 Heavy Metal Toxicity. Life Extension web page. URL: www.lef.org/protocols/prtcls-txt/t-prtcl-156.html. Accessed: Apr 23, 2004.

29 O'Brian J. Mercury Amalgam Toxicity: Your next visit to the dentist may not be as innocent as you think. *Life Extension Magazine.* May 2001.

CHAPTER 2

1 Lindberg S, et al. Group Report: Mercury. In: Hutchison TW, Meemz KM eds. *Lead, Mercury, Cadmium and Arsenic in the Environment.* New York, NY: John Wiley & Sons; 1987.

2 International Programme on Chemical Safety. Environmental Health Criteria 118: Inorganic Mercury. Geneva: World Health Organization (WHO); 1991.

3 Dean RB, et al. The risk to health of chemicals in sewage sludge applied to land. *Waste Manage and Res.* 1985;3:251-278.

4 World Health Organization. Environmental Health Criteria 101: Methylmercury. Geneva: World Health Organization (WHO); 1990.

5 Windham B. Mercury Exposure Levels from Amalgam Dental Fillings:... URL: http://www.home.earthlink.net/berniw1/amalg6.html. Accessed April 14, 2004.

6 International Programme on Chemical Safety. Environmental Health Criteria 118: Inorganic Mercury. Geneva: World Health Organization (WHO); 1991.

7 World Health Organization. Environmental Health Criteria 1: Mercury. Geneva: World Health Organization (WHO); 1990.

8 United States Environmental Protection Agency. Mercury Health Effects Update. Final Report. EPA-600/8-84-019F. 1984.

9 Gay DD, et al. Chewing releases mercury from fillings. *Lancet.* 1979;1(8123):985-986.

10 Svare CW, et al. The effect of dental amalgams on mercury levels in expired air. *J Dent Res.* 1981;60(9):1668-1671.

11 Moller B. Reaction of the human dental pulp to silver amalgam restorations.... *Swed Dent J.* 1978;2(3):93-97.

12 Null, G. Mercury Dental Amalgams - Analyzing the Debate. Dr. Gary Null's webpage on dental Mercury amalgams. URL: http://www.garynull.com/documents/dental/malgam/Amalgam2.htm. Accessed May 5, 2004.

13 World Health Organization. Environmental Health Criteria 101: Methylmercury. Geneva: World Health Organization (WHO); 1990. Geneva.

Chapter 3

1 Diner B. Toxicity, Mercury. emedicine web page. Available at http://www.emedicine.com/emerg/topic813.htm. Accessed Apr 4, 2004.

2 Ibid.

3 International Programme on Chemical Safety. Environmental Health Criteria 118: Inorganic Mercury. World Health Organization, Geneva, 1991.

4 Sehnert K, et al. Is Mercury Toxicity and Autoimmune Disorder? URL: http://www.thorne.com/townsend/oct/mercury.html. Accessed Apr 4, 2004.

5 Hultman P, et al. Adverse immunological effects and autoimmunity induced by dental amalgam and alloy in mice. *FASEB J.* 1994;8(14):1183-1190.

6 Bartova J, et al. Dental amalgam as one of the risk factors in autoimmune diseases. *Neuroendocrinol Lett.* 2003;24(1-2):65-67.

7 Enestrom S, et al. Does amalgam affect the immune system? A controversial issue. *Int Arch Allergy Immunol.* 1995;106(3):180-203.

8 Bagenstose LM, et al. Murine mercury-induced autoimmunity: a model of chemically related autoimmunity in humans. *Immunol Res.* 1999;20(1):67-78.

9 Kim SH, et al. Oral exposure to inorganic mercury alters T lymphocyte phenotypes and cytokine expression in BALB/c mice. *Arch Toxicol.* 2003;77(11):613-620.

10 International Academy of Oral Medicine and Toxicology (IAOMT). A Scientific Response to the American Dental Association's Special Report.... URL: http://www.iaomt.org//documents/A%20Scientific%20Response.pdf. Accessed Aug 3, 2004.

11 Sehnert KW. Autoimmune Disorders. *Advance*, January 1995, pp 47-48.

Chapter 4

1 World Health Organization (WHO). Elemental Mercury and Inorganic Mercury Compounds: Human Health Aspects. URL: http://www.who.int/pcs/cicad/full_text/cicad50.pdf. Accessed June 19, 2004

2 Occupational Safety and Health Administration. Occupational Safety and Health Guideline for Mercury Vapor. URL: http://www.osha.gov/SLTC/healthguidelines/mercuryvapor/recognition.html. Accessed Jun 19. 2004.

3 Ibid.

4 Agency for Toxic Substances and Disease Directory. Minimal Risk Levels (MRLs) for Hazardous Substances. URL: http://www.atsdr.cdc.gov/mrls.html. Accessed Jun 19, 2004.

5 Ibid.

6 World Health Organization (WHO). Elemental Mercury and Inorganic Mercury Compounds: Human Health Aspects. URL: http://www.who.int/pcs/cicad/full_text/cicad50.pdf. Accessed June 19, 2004.

7 Windham B. Facts about Mercury and Dental Amalgam. URL: http://www.eatingalive.com/windham/windhamA.htm. Accessed Apr 14, 2004.

8 National Institute for Occupational Safety and Health (NIOSH). A Recommended Standard for Occupational Exposure to Inorganic Mercury. Published by NTTS PB-222 223, 1973.

CHAPTER 5

1 Dental Amalgam Stirs Controversy. Dr. Doi's Talking Story. Available at: http://www.dentist-doi.com/fall98.htm. Accessed Aug 3, 2004.

2 Mercury and Compounds. U.S. Environmental Protection Agency Web site. Available at: http://www.epa.gov/opptintr/pbt/mercury.htm. Accessed Aug 3, 2004.

3 Null, G. Mercury Dental Amalgams - Analyzing the Debate. Dr. Gary Null's webpage on dental Mercury amalgams. URL: http://www.garynull.com/documents/dental/malgam/Amalgam2.htm. Accessed May 5, 2004.

4 San Francisco Public Utilities Commission. Dental Amalgam Reduction Program Overview http://sfwater.org/detail.cfm/MSC_ID/85/MTO_ID/NULL/MC_ID/4/C_ID/1646/holdSessi on/1#. Accessed June 20, 2004.

5 King County, Natural Resources and Parks, Wastewater Treatment Division. King County regula-tions for dental wastewater discharged to the sewer. http://dnr.metrokc.gov/wlr/indwaste/den-tists.htm. Accessed June 20, 2004.

6 Toronto Municipal Code, Sewers. http://www.city.toronto.on.ca/legdocs/muni-code/1184_681.pdf. Accessed June 20, 2004.

7 Capital Regional District. Sewer Use Bylaw No. 5, 2001 http://www.crd.bc.ca/bylaws/liquid-wastesept_1/bl29229999/bl29229999.pdf. Accessed June 20, 2004.

8 Bio-Probe Newsletter. Amalgam Warning by Manufacturer - March 1998. Bio-Probe Web site. Available at: http://www.bioprobe.com/newsletter/article.asp?article_id=16. Accessed Jul 17,2004.

9 Ibid.

10 Ibid.

11 Ibid.

12 Null, G. Mercury Dental Amalgams - Analyzing the Debate. Dr. Gary Null's webpage on dental Mercury amalgams. URL: http://www.garynull.com/documents/dental/malgam/Amalgam2.htm. Accessed May 5, 2004.

13 Press Release. Iowa First to Ban Mercury from Childhood Vaccines. URL: http://www.universi-tyofhealth.net/PR/051604PressRelease1stHgLawIA.htm. Accessed Jun 6, 2004.

14 Lohyn R, et al. ASOMAT [Australasian Society of Oral Medicine and Toxicology] submission to amalgam review working party [of Australia's National Health and Medical Research Council], Part B. May 1988; p50.

15 Ibid.

16 Newspaper article. *Svenska Dagblodet*. May 20, 1987. as cited in Null, G. Mercury Dental Amalgams - Analyzing the Debate. URL: http://www.garynull.com/documents/dental/malgam/Amalgam2.htm. Accessed May 5, 2004.

17 Chua J, et al. Special Reports: Mercury in the Mouth - the Debate over Dental Amalgams. CBC News webpage. URL: http://www.cbc.ca/consumers/indepth/mercury/index.html. Accessed Jun 6, 2004.

18 Wyndham B. Documentation of Adverse Effects. URL: http://www.home.earthlink.net/~berniew1/. Accessed June 20, 2004.

19 Dodes JE. The amalgam controversy. An evidence-based analysis. *J Am Dent Assoc.* 2001;132(3):348-356.

CHAPTER 6

1 O'Brian J. Mercury Amalgam Toxicity: Your next visit to the dentist may not be as innocent as you think. *Life Extension Magazine.* May 2001.

2 Ahlqwist M, et al. Number of amalgam tooth fillings in relation to subjectively experienced symptoms in a study of Swedish women. *Community Dent Oral Epidemiol.* 1988;16(4):227-231.

3 Yip HK, et al. Dental amalgam and human health. *Int Dent J.* 2003;53(6):464-468.

4 Dodes JE. The amalgam controversy. An evidence-based analysis. *J Am Dent Assoc.* 2001;132(3):348-356.

5 Saxe SR, et al. Alzheimer's disease, dental amalgam and mercury. *J Am Dent Assoc.* 1999;130(2):191-199.

6 Bengtsson C, et al. [No connection between the number of amalgam fillings and health. Epidemiological observations from a population study of women in Gothenburg]. *Lakartidningen.* 2001;98(9):930-933.

7 Brune D. Corrosion of amalgams. *Scand J Dent Res.* 1981;89(6):506-514.

8 Brune D, et al. Man's mercury loading from a dental amalgam. *Sci Total Environ.* 1985;44(1):51-63.

9 Gay DD, et al. Chewing releases mercury from fillings. *Lancet.* 1979;1(8123):985-986.

10 Svare CW, et al. The effect of dental amalgams on mercury levels in expired air. *J Dent Res.* 1981;60(9):1668-1671.

11 Abraham JE, et al. The effect of dental amalgam restorations on blood mercury levels. *J Dent Res.* 1984;63(1):71-73.

12 Vimy MJ, et al. Estimation of mercury body burden from dental amalgam: computer simulation of a metabolic compartmental model. *J Dent Res.* 1986;65(12):1415-1419.

13 Abraham JE, et al. The effect of dental amalgam restorations on blood mercury levels. *J Dent Res.* 1984;63(1):71-73.

14 Vimy MJ, et al. Serial measurements of intra-oral air mercury: estimation of daily dose from dental amalgam. *J Dent Res.* 1985;64(8):1072-1075.

15 Enwonwu CO. Potential health hazard of use of mercury in dentistry: critical review of the literature. *Environ Res.* 1987;42(1):257-274.

16 Friberg L, et al. [The release and uptake of metallic mercury vapour from amalgam.] In: Mercury/amalgam - health risks. Report by an expert group. Stockholm: National Board of Health and Welfare, Report series *Socialstyrelsen Redovisar.* 1987;10:65-79.

17 World Health Organization (WHO). Elemental Mercury and Inorganic Mercury Compounds: Human Health Aspects. URL: http://www.who.int/pcs/cicad/full_text/cicad50.pdf. Accessed June 19, 2004.

18 Vimy MJ, et al. Serial measurements of intra-oral air mercury: estimation of daily dose from dental amalgam. *J Dent Res.* 1985;64(8):1072-1075.

19 Nylander M, et al. Mercury concentrations in the human brain and kidneys in relation to exposure from dental amalgam fillings. *Swed Dent J.* 1987;11(5):179-187.

20 Nylander M, et al. Mercury accumulation in tissues from dental staff and controls in relation to exposure. *Swed Dent J.* 1989;13(6):235-243.

21 Eggleston DW, et al. Correlation of dental amalgam with mercury in brain tissue. *J Prosthet Dent.* 1987;58(6):704-707.

22 World Health Organization (WHO). Elemental Mercury and Inorganic Mercury Compounds: Human Health Aspects. URL: http://www.who.int/pcs/cicad/full_text/cicad50.pdf. Accessed June 19, 2004.

23 Hahn LJ, et al. Dental "silver" tooth fillings: a source of mercury exposure revealed by whole-body image scan and tissue analysis. *FASEB J.* 1989;3(14):2641-2646.

24 Vimy MJ, et al. Maternal-fetal distribution of mercury (203Hg) released from dental amalgam fillings. *Am J Physiol.* 1990;258(4 Pt 2):R939-R945.

25 International Academy of Oral Medicine and Toxicology (IAOMT). A Scientific Response to the American Dental Association's Special Report.... URL: http://www.iaomt.org//documents/A%20Scientific%20Response.pdf Accessed Aug 3, 2004.

26 Vimy MJ, et al. Mercury from maternal "silver" tooth fillings in sheep and human breast milk. A source of neonatal exposure. *Biol Trace Elem Res.* 1997;56(2):143-152.

27 Snapp KR, et al. The contribution of dental amalgam to mercury in blood. *J Dent Res.* 1989;68(5):780-785.

28 Molin M, et al. Mercury, selenium, and glutathione peroxidase before and after amalgam removal in man. *Acta Odontol Scand.* 1990;48(3):189-202.

29 Sandborgh-Englund G, et al. Mercury in biological fluids after amalgam removal. *J Dent Res.* 1998;77(4):615-624.

30 Bjorkman L, et al. Mercury in saliva and feces after removal of amalgam fillings. *Toxicol Appl Pharmacol.* 1997;144(1):156-162.

31 Berglund A, et al. Mercury levels in plasma and urine after removal of all amalgam restorations: the effect of using rubber dams. *Dent Mater.* 1997;13(5):297-304.

32 Malmström C, et al. Silver amalgam: An unstable material. *Danish Dental Journal. Tidsskr. f. Tandlaeger.* October 1989. Swedish paper translated by Mats Hansson Ph.D., in *Bio-Probe Newsletter,* Vol 9(1):5-6, Jan. 1993.

CHAPTER 7

1 Null, G. Mercury Dental Amalgams - Analyzing the Debate. Dr. Gary Null's webpage on dental Mercury amalgams. URL: http://www.garynull.com/documents/dental/malgam/Amalgam2.htm. Accessed May 5, 2004.

2 Ibid.

3 Watson DE. Consumer Choice and Implementing Full disclosure in Dentistry - Opening Remarks of Diane E. Watson, M.C. Human Rights and Wellness Hearing, Washington DC. May 8th, 2003. URL: http://reform.house.gov/UploadedFiles/Diane%20Watson%20opening%20statement.pdf. Accessed July 04, 2004.

4 Dentists' Frequently Asked Questions about Proposition 65. California Dental Association web page. URL: http://www.cda.019/member/news/prop65faq.htm. Accessed Apr 19, 2004.

5 International Programme on Chemical Safety. Environmental Health Criteria 118: Inorganic Mercury. Geneva: World Health Organization (WHO); 1991.

6 Centers for Disease Control and Prevention (CDC). Morbidity & Mortality Weekly Report (MMWR). March 02, 2001. 50(08);140-3.

7 von Muhlendahl KE. [The toxicity of mercury in amalgam dental fillings]. *Padiatr Grenzgeb*. 1992;31(1) :21-25.

8 Kazantzis G. Mercury exposure and early effects: an overview. *Med Lav*. 2002;93(3):139-147.

9 Lien DC, et al. Accidental inhalation of mercury vapour: respiratory and toxicologic consequences. *Can Med Assoc J*. 1983;129(6):591-595.

10 Stoz F, et al. [Is a generalized amalgam ban justified? Studies of mothers and their newborn infants]. *Z Geburtshilfe Perinatol*. 1995;199(1):35-41.

11 Jauniaux E, et al. Distribution and transfer pathways of antioxidant molecules inside the first trimester human gestational sac. *J Clin Endocrinol Metab*. 2004 Mar;89(3):1452-8.

12 Vimy MJ, et al.. Maternal-fetal distribution of mercury (203Hg) released from dental amalgam fillings. *Am J Physiol*. 1990;258(4 Pt 2):R939-R945.

13 O'Brian J. Mercury Amalgam Toxicity: Your next visit to the dentist may not be as innocent as you think. *Life Extension Magazine*. May 2001.

14 Heavy Metal Toxicity. Life Extension web page. URL: www.lef.org/protocols/prtcls-txt/t-prtcl-156.html. Accessed: Apr 23, 2004.

15 O'Brian J. Mercury Amalgam Toxicity: Your next visit to the dentist may not be as innocent as you think. *Life Extension Magazine*. May 2001.

16 Ariza ME, et al. Mutagenesis of AS52 cells by low concentrations of lead (II) and mercury (II). *Environ Mol Mutagen*. 1996;27(1):30-3.

17 Bahia Mde O, et al. Genotoxic effects of mercury on in vitro cultures of human cells. *An Acad Bras Cienc*. 1999;71(3 Pt 1):437-43.

18 Elghany NA, et al. Occupational exposure to inorganic mercury vapour and reproductive outcomes. *Occup Med (Lond)*. 1997 Aug;47(6):333-6.

19 Boadi WY, et al. In vitro effect of mercury on enzyme activities and its accumulation in the first-trimester human placenta. *Environ Res*. 1992; Feb;57(1):96-106.

20 Sakamoto M, et al.. Evaluation of changes in methylmercury accumulation in the developing rat brain and its effects.... *Brain Res*. 2002 Sep 13;949(1-2):51-9.

21 Metal Toxicity. Life Extension web page. URL: www.lef.org/protocols/prtcls-txt/t-prtcl-156.html. Accessed: Apr 23, 2004.

22 Schettler T. Toxic threats to neurologic development of children. *Environ Health Perspect*. 2001 Dec;109 Suppl 6:813-6.

23 Mendola P, et al. Environmental factors associated with a spectrum of neurodevelopmental deficits. *Ment Retard Dev Disabil Res Rev*. 2002;8(3):188-97.

24 Bernard S, et al. The role of mercury in the pathogenesis of autism. *Mol Psychiatry*. 2002;7 Suppl 2:S42-3.

25 Heavy Metal Toxicity. Life Extension web page. URL: www.lef.org/protocols/prtcls-txt/t-prtcl-156.html. Accessed: Apr 23, 2004.

26 The Children's Amalgam Trial: design and methods. *Control Clin Trials*. 2003;24(6):795-814.

27 Vimy MJ, et al. Maternal-fetal distribution of mercury (203Hg) released from dental amalgam fillings. *Am J Physiol*. 1990 Apr;258(4 Pt 2):R939-45.

28 Marsh DO, et al. Fetal methylmercury poisoning: clinical and toxicological data on 29 cases. *Ann Neurol*. 1980;7(4):348-353.

29 Eyl TB. Methyl mercury poisoning in fish and human beings. *Clin Toxicol*. 1971;4(2):291-296.

30 Vahter M, et al. Longitudinal study of methylmercury and inorganic mercury in blood and urine of pregnant and lactating women, as well as in umbilical cord blood. *Environ Res*. 2000;84(2):186-194.

31 Holmes AS, et al. Reduced levels of mercury in first baby haircuts of autistic children. *Int J Toxicol*. 2003 Jul-Aug; 22(4):277-85.

32 Vahter M, et al. Longitudinal study of methylmercury and inorganic mercury in blood and urine of pregnant and lactating women, as well as in umbilical cord blood. *Environ Res*. 2000 Oct;84(2):186-94.

33 Drasch G, et al. Mercury in human colostrum and early breast milk. Its dependence on dental amalgam and other factors. *J Trace Elem Med Biol*. 1998 Mar;12(1):23-7.

34 Vimy MJ, et al. Mercury from maternal "silver" tooth fillings in sheep and human breast milk. A source of neonatal exposure. *Biol Trace Elem Res*. 1997 Feb;56(2):143-52.

35 Schulte A, et al. [Mercury concentrations in the urine of children with and without amalgam fillings]. *Schweiz Monatsschr Zahnmed*. 1994;104(11):1336-1340.

36 Kordi-Mood M, et al. Urinary mercury excretion following amalgam filling in children. *J Toxicol. Clin Toxicol*. 2001;39(7):701-705.

37 Gabrio T, et al. [10 years of observation by public health offices in Baden-Wurttemberg-assessment of human biomonitoring for mercury due to dental amalgam fillings and other sources]. *Gesundheitswesen*. 2003;65(5):327-335.

38 Khordi-Mood M, et al. Urinary mercury excretion following amalgam filling in children. *J Toxicol Clin Toxicol*. 2001;39(7):701-705.

39 Null, G. Mercury Dental Amalgams - Analyzing the Debate. Dr. Gary Null's webpage on dental Mercury amalgams. URL: http://www.garynull.com/documents/dental/malgam/Amalgam2.htm. Accessed May 5, 2004.

40 Mercury in Vaccines and an Increase in Autism. Thimerosal information resource. http://www.thimerosal-legal.com. Accessed July 13, 2004.

CHAPTER 8

1 Chang LW, et al. Blood-brain barrier dysfunction in experimental mercury intoxication. *Acta Neuropathol (Berl)* 1972;21(3):179-84.

2 Haley BE. *Dr. Boyd E Haley Responds to Robert M. Anderton DDS, President of the ADA*. Washington, DC. Committee on Government Reform. U.S. House of Representatives, 2001.

3 Windham B. Dental Amalgam Fillings Page. Available at:

http://www.earthlink.net~berniew1/indexa.html. Accessed April 14, 2004.

4 Hussain S, et al. Mercuric chloride-induced reactive oxygen species and its effect on antioxidant enzymes in different regions of rat brain. *J Environ Sci Health B* 1997 May;32(3):395-409.

5 Perrin-Nadif R, et al. Catalase and superoxide dismutase activities as biomarkers of oxidative stress in workers exposed to mercury vapors. *J Toxicol Environ Health* 1996 June 7;48(2):107-19.

6 Quig D. Cysteine metabolism and metal toxicity. *Altern Med Rev* 1998 August;3(4):262-70.

7 Zabinski Z, et al. The activity of erythrocyte enzymes and basic indices of peripheral blood erythrocytes from workers chronically exposed to mercury vapours. *Toxicol Ind Health* 2000 February;16(2):58-64.

8 Shenker BJ, et al. Immunotoxic effects of mercuric compounds on human lymphocytes and monocytes. II. Alterations in cell viability. *Immunopharmacol Immunotoxicol* 1992;14(3):555-77.

9 Eggleston DW. Effect of dental amalgam and nickel alloys on T-lymphocytes: preliminary report. *J Prosthet Dent* 1984 May;51(5):617-23.

10 Perlingeiro RC, et al. Polymorphonuclear phagocytosis and killing in workers exposed to inorganic mercury. *Int J Immunopharmacol* 1994 December;16(12):1011-7.

11 Christensen MM, et al. Influence of mercuric chloride on resistance to generalized infection with herpes simplex virus type 2 in mice. *Toxicology* 1996 November 15;114(1):57-66.

12 Omura Y, et al. Role of mercury (Hg) in resistant infections & effective treatment of Chlamydia trachomatis and Herpes family viral infections.... *Acupunct Electrother Res* 1995 August;20(3-4):195-229.

13 Christensen MM, et al. Influence of mercuric chloride on resistance to generalized infection with herpes simplex virus type 2 in mice.*Toxicology*. 1996 Nov 15;114(1):57-66.

14 Windham B. Dental Amalgam Fillings Page. URL: http://www.earthlink.net~berniew1/indexa.html. Accessed April 14, 2004.

15 Mathieson PW. Mercury: God of TH2 cells. *Clin Exp Immunol.* Nov 1995; 102(2): 229-230

16 Bangentose LM et al. Mercury induced autoimmunity in humans *Immunol Res.* 1999;20(1): 67-78.

17 Shenker BJ, et al. Immunotoxic effects of mercuric compounds on human lymphocytes and monocytes. II. Alterations in cell viability. *Immunopharmacol Immunotoxicol* 1992;14(3):555-77.

18 Hultman P, et al. Adverse immunological effects and autoimmunity induced by dental amalgam and alloy in mice. *FASEB J* 1994 November;8(14):1183-90.

19 Sehnert K, et al. Is Mercury Toxicity an Auto-immune Disorder? URL: http://www.thorne.com/townsend/oct/mercury.html. Accessed April 04, 2004.

20 Miszta H, et al. Effect of mercury and combined effect of mercury and dimethylsulphoxide (DMSO).... *Folia Haematol Int Mag Klin Morphol Blutforsch* 1989;116(1):151-5.

21 Silberud R. Report of the International Conference on the Biocompatability of Materials. Colorado State University, 1998.

22 Ibid.

23 Ronnback L, et al. Chronic encephalopathies induced by mercury or lead: aspects of underlying cellular and molecular mechanisms. *Br J Ind Med.* 1992 Apr;49(4):233-40.

24 Walum E, et al. Use of primary cultures and continuous cell lines to study effects on astrocytic

regulatory functions. *Clin Exp Pharmacol Physiol.* 1995 Apr;22(4):284-7.

25 Mader S. *Inquiry into Life* - 10th edition. New York, NY: McGraw-Hill; 2003.

26 Clauw DJ. The pathogenesis of chronic pain and fatigue syndromes, with special reference to fibromyalgia. *Med Hypotheses.* 1995 May;44(5):369-78.

27 Pendergrass JC, et al. The Toxic Effects of Mercury on CNS Proteins - Similarity to Observations in Alzheimer's Disease. IAOMT Symposium paper. March, 1997.

28 Leong CC, et al. Retrograde degeneration of neurite membrane structural integrity of nerve growth cones following in vitro exposure to mercury. *Neuroreport.* 2001;12(4):733-737.

29 Olivieri G, et al. Mercury induces cell cytotoxicity and oxidative stress and increases beta-amyloid secretion and tau phosphorylation in SHSY5Y neuroblastoma cells. *J Neurochem.* 2000 January;74(1):231-6.

30 Thompson CM, et al. Regional brain trace-element studies in Alzheimer's disease. *Neurotoxicology.* 1988 Spring;9(1):1-7.

31 Windham B. Dental Amalgam Fillings Page. Available at: http://www.earthlink.net~berniew1/indexa.html. Accessed April 14, 2004.

32 Pendergrass JC, et al. Mercury vapor inhalation inhibits binding of GTP to tubulin in rat brain: similarity to a molecular lesion in Alzheimer diseased brain. *Neurotoxicology.* 1997;18(2):315-24.

33 Quicksilver Associates. *The mercury in your mouth*, p 60, as cited in Null G. Mercury dental amalgams analysing the debate. Available at: http://www.garynull.com/documents/dental/amalgam/Amalgam2.htm. Accessed May 5, 2004.

CHAPTER 9

1 Duke RC, et al. Cell suicide in health and disease. *Sci Am* 1996 December;275(6):80-7.

2 Slater AF et al. Signalling mechanisms and oxidative stress in apoptosis. *Toxicol Lett* 1995 December;82-83:149-53

3 Kidd PM. Glutathione: Systemic Protectant Against Oxidative and Free Radical Damage. 2004. URL: http://www.thorne.com/altmedrev/fulltext/glut.html. Accessed February 7, 2004.

4 MacWilliam LD. Glutathione. In: *Comparative Guide to Nutritional Supplements.* Vernon, BC. Northern Dimensions Publishing. 2003: 44-47.

5 Kerper LE, et al., Ballatori N. Methylmercury efflux from brain capillary endothelial cells is modulated by intracellular glutathione but not ATP. *Toxicol Appl Pharmacol.* 1996;141(2):526-531.

6 Fujiyama J, et al. Mechanism of methylmercury efflux from cultured astrocytes. *Biochem Pharmacol.* 1994;47(9):1525-1530.

7 Droge W, et al. Functions of glutathione and glutathione disulfide in immunology and immunopathology. *FASEB J.* 1994;8(14):1131-1138.

8 Fidelus RK, et al. Glutathione and lymphocyte activation: a function of aging and auto-immune disease. *Immunology* 1987 August;61(4):503-8.

9 Anderson ME. Glutathione and glutathione delivery compounds. Adv Pharmacol. 1997;38: 65-78.

10 Droge W, et al. Role of cysteine and glutathione in HIV infection and cancer cachexia: therapeutic

intervention with N-acetylcysteine. *Adv Pharmacol.* 1997;38:581-600.

11 Lee YW, et al. Role of reactive oxygen species and glutathione in inorganic mercury- induced injury in human glioma cells. *Neurochem Res.* 2001;26(11):1187-1193.

12 Lohr JB, et al. Free Radical Involvement in Neuropsychiatric Illnesses. *Psychopharmacol Bull.* 1995;31(1):159-165.

13 Jenner P. Oxidative damage in neurodegenerativeneurological disease. *Lancet.* 1994;344(8925): 796-798.

14 Zalups RK. Molecular interactions with mercury in the kidney. *Pharmacol Rev.* 2000;52(1):113-143.

15 Kromidas L, et al. The protective effects of glutathione against methylmercury cytotoxicity. *Toxicol Lett.* 1990;51(1):67-80.

16 Patrick L. Mercury toxicity and antioxidants: Part I: role of glutathione and alpha-lipoic acid in the treatment of mercury toxicity. *Altern Med Rev.* 2002;7(6):456-471.

17 Horrobin DF. Multiple sclerosis: the rational basis for treatment with colchicine and evening primrose oil. *Med Hypotheses.* 1979;5(3):365-378.

18 Johnston CS, et al. Vitamin C elevates red blood cell glutathione in healthy adults. *Am J Clin Nutr.* 1993;58(1):103-105.

19 Lomaestro BM, et al. Glutathione in health and disease: pharmacotherapeutic issues.." *Ann Pharmacother.* 1995;29(12):1263-1273.

20 Tateishi N, et al. Relative contributions of sulfur atoms of dietary cysteine and methionine to rat liver glutathione and proteins. *J Biochem (Tokyo).* 1981;90(6):1603-1610.

21 Patrick L. Mercury toxicity and antioxidants: Part I: role of glutathione and alpha-lipoic acid in the treatment of mercury toxicity. *Altern Med Rev.* 2002;7(6):456-471.

22 Han D, et al. Lipoic acid increases de novo synthesis of cellular glutathione by improving cystine utilization. *Biofactors.* 1997;6(3):321-338.

23 Gregus Z, et al. Effect of lipoic acid on biliary excretion of glutathione and metals. *Toxicol Appl Pharmacol.* 1992;114(1):88-96.

24 MacWilliam LD. Glutathione. In: *Comparative Guide to Nutritional Supplements.* Vernon, BC. Northern Dimensions Publishing. 2003: 44-47.

CHAPTER 10

1 DAMS Inc. *Mercury Free and Healthy, The Dental Amalgam Issue.* DAMS Inc., along with Consumers for Dental Choice. A Project of the National Institute for Science, Law and Public Policy. Washington, DC, 20036.

2 Lister RE. Mercury and Selenium - the Battle of the Elements. *Complementary Health Magazine online.* URL: www.postivehealth.com/permit/Articles/Dentist/lister7.htm. Accessed Jun 5, 2004.

3 Richards JM et al. Mercury vapour released during the removal of old amalgam restorations. Br Dent J. 1985 Oct 5;159(7):231-2.

4 Windham B. Mercury Exposure Levels from Amalgam Dental Fillings.... URL: http://www.home.earthlink.net/berniw1/amalg6.html. Accessed April 14, 2004.

5 Aposhian HV. Mobilization of mercury and arsenic in humans by sodium 2,3-dimercapto-1-propane sulfonate (DMPS). *Environ Health Perspect*. 1998 Aug;106 Suppl 4:1017-25.

6 Gonzalez-Ramirez D, et al. Sodium 2,3-dimercaptopropane-1-sulfonate challenge test for mercury in humans: II.... *J Pharmacol Exp Ther*. 1995 Jan;272(1):264-74.

7 Echeverria D, et al. Neurobehavioral effects from exposure to dental amalgam Hg(o): new distinctions between recent exposure and Hg body burden. *FASEB J*. 1998 Aug;12(11):971-80.

8 Akesson I. Status of mercury and selenium in dental personnel: impact of amalgam work and own fillings. *Arch Environ Health*. 1991 Mar-Apr;46(2):102-9.

9 Windham B. Mercury Exposure Levels from Amalgam Dental Fillings.... URL: http://www.home.earthlink.net/berniw1/amalg6.html. Accessed April 14, 2004.

10 Agency for Toxic Substances and Disease Registry. *Minimal Risk Levels (MRLs) for Hazardous Substances*. URL: http://www.atsdr.cdc.gov/mrls.html. Accessed Jun 14, 2004

11 Nylander M, et al. Mercury accumulation in tissues from dental staff and controls in relation to exposure. *Swed Dent J*. 1989;13(6):235-43.

12 International Programme on Chemical Safety. Environmental Health Criteria 118: Inorganic Mercury. Geneva: World Health Organization (WHO); 1991.

13 O'Brian J. Mercury Amalgam Toxicity: Your next visit to the dentist may not be as innocent as you think. *Life Extension Magazine*. May 2001.

14 Moller AT, et al. Stress and coping amongst South African dentists in private practice. *J Dent Assoc S Afr*. 1996 Jun;51(6):347-57.

15 Echeverria D, et al. Neurobehavioral effects from exposure to dental amalgam Hg(o): new distinctions between recent exposure and Hg body burden. FASEB J. 1998 Aug;12(11):971-80.

16 Windham B. Mercury Exposure Levels from Amalgam Dental Fillings: Documentation of Mechanisms by Which Mercury Causes over 30 Chronic Health Conditions. URL: http://www.home.earthlink.net/berniw1/amalg6.html. Accessed April 14, 2004.

17 Rowland AS, et al. The effect of occupational exposure to mercury vapour on the fertility of female dental assistants. Occup Environ Med. 1994 Jan;51(1):28-34.

18 Cordier S, et al. Paternal exposure to mercury and spontaneous abortions. Br J Ind Med. 1991 Jun;48(6):375-81.

19 Windham B. Mercury Exposure Levels from Amalgam Dental Fillings.... URL: http://www.home.earthlink.net/berniw1/amalg6.html. Accessed April 14, 2004.

CHAPTER 11

1 Huggins H. Medical and Legal Implications of Components of Dental Amalgams. As cited in: Null, G. Mercury Dental Amalgams - Analyzing the Debate. URL: www.garynull.com/documents/dental/amalgam/Amalgam2.htm. Accessed May 19, 2004.

2 Toxic Research Foundation. Micromercurialism: Environment and Responsibility. July 1987. As cited in: Null, G. Mercury Dental Amalgams - Analyzing the Debate. URL: www.garynull.com/documents/dental/amalgam/Amalgam2.htm. Accessed May 19, 2004.

3 Stortebacker P. Direct Transport of Mercury from the Oro-nasal Cavity to the Cranial Cavity as a Cause of Dental Amalgam Poisoning. *Swed J Biologic Med*. March, 1980:19.

4 Bengtsson U. On the Stability of Amalgams. On Reality - Images, Experiences, and Distortions. URL: http://www.gbg.bonet.se/bwf/art/instab/formation.html. Accessed July 4, 2004.

5 Huggins H. Medical and Legal Implications of Components of Dental Amalgams. As cited in: Null, G. Mercury Dental Amalgams - Analyzing the Debate. URL: www.garynull.com/documents/dental/amalgam/Amalgam2.htm. Accessed May 19, 2004.

6 Svare CW, et al. The effect of dental amalgams on mercury levels in expired air. *J Dent Res.* 1981;60(9):1668-1671.

7 Vimy MJ, et al. Intra-oral air mercury released from dental amalgam. *J Dent Res.* 1985 Aug; 64(8):1069-71.

8 Ibid.

9 Patterson JE, et al. Mercury in human breath from dental amalgams. *Bull Environ Contam Toxicol.* 1985;34(4):459-468.

10 Malmström C, et al. Silver amalgam: An unstable material. *Danish Dental Journal. Tidsskr. f. Tandlaeger.* October 1989. Swedish paper translated by Mats Hansson Ph.D., in *Bio-Probe Newsletter,* Vol 9(1):5-6, Jan.1993.

11 Huggins HA, et al. *Uniformed Consent: the Hidden Dangers in Dental Care.* Charlottesvilee, VA: Hampton Roads Publishing Company Inc; 1999.

12 Olsson S, et al. Release of elements due to electrochemical corrosion of dental amalgam. *J Dent Res.* 1994;73(1):33-43.

13 Windham B. Dental Fillings page. URL: http//:www.earthlink.net/~berniew1/amalg6.html. Accessed on Mar 14, 2004.

CHAPTER 14

1 Engel P.[Observations on health before and after amalgam removal] *Schweiz Monatsschr Zahnmed.* 1998;108(8):811-3. German.

2 Kidd RF. Results of dental amalgam removal and mercury detoxification using DMPS and neural therapy. *Altern Ther Health Med.* 2000 Jul;6(4):49-55.

3 Sandborgh-Englund G, et al. Mercury in biological fluids after amalgam removal. *J Dent Res.* 1998 Apr;77(4):615-24.

4 Berglund A, et al. Mercury levels in plasma and urine after removal of all amalgam restorations: the effect of using rubber dams. *Dent Mater.* 1997 Sep;13(5):297-304.

5 Bergerow J, et al. Long-term mercury excretion in the urine after removal of amalgam fillings. *Int Arch Occup Environ Health.* 1994;66(3):209-212.

6 Snapp KR, et al. The contribution of dental amalgam to mercury in blood. *J Dent Res.* 1989 May;68(5):780-5.

7 Molin M, et al. Mercury, selenium, and glutathione peroxidase before and after amalgam removal in man. *Acta Odontol Scand.* 1990 Jun;48(3):189-202.

8 Sandborgh-Englund G, et al. Mercury in biological fluids after amalgam removal. *J Dent Res.* 1998 Apr;77(4):615-24.

9 Bjorkman L, et al. Mercury in saliva and feces after removal of amalgam fillings. *Toxicol Appl Pharmacol.* 1997 May;144(1):156-62.

10 Jones L. Dental Amalgam and Health Experience: Exploring Health Outcomes and Issues for People Medically Diagnosed with Mercury Poisoning. *Bulletin of the New Zealand Psychological Society.* 1999;97:29-33.

11 Lindh U, et al. Removal of dental amalgam and other metal alloys supported by antioxidant therapy.... *Neuroendocrinol Lett.* 2002 Oct-Dec;23(5-6):459-82.

12 DAMS Inc. The Dental Amalgam Issue. *Mercury Free and Healthy* web page. URL: www.amalgam.org. Accessed July 4, 2004.

CHAPTER 15

1 American Dental Association. ADA Positions and Statements: ADA Statement on Dental Amalgam, Jan 8, 2002. URL: www.ada.org/prof/resources/positions/statements/amalgam.asp. Accessed Jun 12, 2004.

2 International Academy of Oral Medicine and Toxicology (IAOMT). A Scientific Response to the American Dental Association's Special Report.... URL: http://www.iaomt.org//documents/A%20Scientific%20Response.pdf. Accessed Aug 3, 2004.

3 Galic N, et al. Dental amalgam mercury exposure in rats. *Biometals.* 1999 Sep;12(3):227-31

4 Null G. Mercury Dental Amalgams - Analyzing the Debate. Gary Null's Natural Living Web site. URL: http://www.garynull.com. Accessed Jun 6, 2004.

5 Dental Amalgam Fillings the Number One Source of Mercury in People. Positive Health Magazine web page. URL: http://www.positivehealth.com/permit/Articles/Dentist/dental.htm. Accessed Jun 12, 2004.

6 Dental Amalgam Fillings the Number One Source of Mercury in People. Positive Health Magazine web page. URL: http://www.positivehealth.com/permit/Articles/Dentist/dental.htm. Accessed Jun 12, 2004.

7 International Academy of Oral Medicine and Toxicology (IAOMT). A Scientific Response to the American Dental Association's Special Report.... URL: http://www.iaomt.org//documents/A%20Scientific%20Response.pdf. Accessed Aug 3, 2004.

8 Ibid.

9 Ibid.

10 Letter to Dr. James Brookfield, President, Canadian Dental Association. Feb 27, 1996.

11 American Dental Association News release, as cited in: Null G. Mercury Dental Amalgams - Analyzing the Debate. Gary Null's Natural Living Web site. URL: http://www.garynull.com. Accessed Jun 6, 2004.